AF802678

Ménière's Disease

Evidence and Outcomes

Ménière's Disease

Evidence and Outcomes

Michael J. Ruckenstein, MD, MSc, FACS, FRCSC

PLURAL PUBLISHING
INC.
SAN DIEGO
OXFORD
BRISBANE

Plural Publishing
Inc.

5521 Ruffin Road
San Diego, CA 92123

e-mail: info@pluralpublishing.com
Web site: http://www.pluralpublishing.com

49 Bath Street
Abingdon, Oxfordshire OX14 1EA
United Kingdom

Copyright © by Plural Publishing, Inc. 2010

Typeset in 10½/13 Palatino by Flanagan's Publishing Services, Inc.
Printed in the United States of America by Bang Printing

All rights, including that of translation, reserved. No part of this publication may be reproduced, stored in a retrieval system, or transmitted in any form or by any means, electronic, mechanical, recording, or otherwise, including photocopying, recording, taping, Web distribution, or information storage and retrieval systems without the prior written consent of the publisher.

For permission to use material from this text, contact us by
Telephone: (866) 758-7251
Fax: (888) 758-7255
e-mail: permissions@pluralpublishing.com

Every attempt has been made to contact the copyright holders for material originally printed in another source. If any have been inadvertently overlooked, the publishers will gladly make the necessary arrangements at the first opportunity.

Library of Congress Cataloging-in-Publication Data

Ruckenstein, Michael J. (Michael Jay), 1960-
Ménière's disease : evidence and outcomes / Michael J. Ruckenstein.
p. ; cm.
Includes bibliographical references and index.
ISBN-13: 978-1-59756-300-0 (alk. paper)
ISBN-10: 1-59756-300-5 (alk. paper)
1. Ménière's disease. I. Title.
[DNLM: 1. Meniere Disease. WV 258 R911m 2010]
RF275.R83 2010
617.8'82—dc22

2010004798

Contents

Introduction

I first made a presentation on Ménière's disease as a medical student in McGill University interested in pursuing a career in otolaryngology. At the time, the subject seemed like an obvious choice as it was one of the few otolaryngologic disorders I was familiar with, as my mother had suffered from Ménière's disease for many years. The literature I reviewed left me very intrigued by the disorder. It seemed to leave many questions unanswered and quite a number of concepts seemed contradictory. I remember that one of my initial observations was questioning why physicians would simultaneously treat the disorder with histamine and an antihistamine! During my initial years of residency at the University of Toronto, I began preparing a Grand Rounds that was designed to explore the treatment of Ménière's disease. As I read papers about treatment of the disorder I became simultaneously more confused, but also more interested. I accumulated hundreds of papers, which caused considerable consternation among my coresidents as they occupied increasingly more space in our call room at the Toronto General Hospital! I ended up presenting two consecutive Grand Rounds on the subject as I had accumulated so much information. I remember Dr. Patrick Gullane sitting in the front row of my presentation nodding and following every word enthusiastically. Part of this was Pat's nature; I knew Pat was always intellectually curious and an enthusiast. Nonetheless, I felt if I could interest a head and neck surgeon of world renown on the subject of the treatment of Ménière's disease, I must be onto something! I have continued what has been a long fascination with the disorder of Ménière's disease, and this book is a byproduct of this intellectual focus.

I feel it is imperative to acknowledge my mentors who have guided and influenced me throughout my career. Drs. Ron Fenton, Julian Nedzelski, and John Rutka had a major influence on me during my residency. I remember sitting in the cafeteria of St. Michael's Hospital listening to Dr. Fenton and absorbing these thoughts on Ménière's disease. Julian Nedzelski, MD has been a true role model and mentor and taught me that a neurotologist can be both an expert in the medical treatment of neurotologic disorders as well as an outstanding skull base surgeon. Perhaps more than anyone, John Rutka, MD provided me with the guidance and insight necessary to critically evaluate the literature. Dr. Robert Harrison, PhD, was my research mentor and continues to be among my closest friends. The auditory neuroscience I learned under his tutelage provided me with the foundation necessary to better understand the literature pertaining to the pathophysiology of the disease. His influence is very much felt in the chapter on pathophysiology. Jeffrey Harris, MD, PhD, my fellowship mentor and supervisor, shares a passion with me pertaining to Ménière's disease. We had many discussions about the disorder, and I carry the insights I gained from him to this day. Dr. Roberto Cueva, my other fellowship supervisor, is an absolutely superb neurotologist and an even finer person. I always considered it an honor and privilege to have been mentored by Bob, and his influence is felt very profoundly in this book, particularly in the chapter pertaining to surgery of the disorder.

In my travels in academic medicine, I have had the privilege of working with absolutely outstanding professionals. A few of those individuals graciously consented to provide chapters for this book, and I would like to thank Drs. Neil Sheppard, PhD and Jeffrey Staab, MD, as well as Elizabeth Grace, PT, MS, NCS for these contributions. Dr. Stephen Rauch is a leading authority on Ménière's disease and I am very grateful to him for contributing a chapter on temporal bone histopathology. Dr. Marc Eisen is a former resident here at the University of Pennsylvania. Those who know Marc consider him to be a brilliant individual with an interest in the history of our subspecialty and I am grateful for his contribution on the subject of the history of Ménière's disease. The reader will notice that many of our Penn residents are coauthors with me of various chapters of this book; my hope was to provide an opportunity to participate in an exercise in critical thinking. I gained much from their fresh insights, and I hope they benefited from the experience.

Judy Meyer, my editor for Plural Publishing, put up with my procrastination and failure to meet many deadlines with a smile and good humor. I am sure she is quite relieved to have this book off her agenda and I do very much appreciate her intelligence and understanding. Without the happiness I derive from my family, none of my academic achievements would hold any meaning. Words cannot express the love and gratitude I hold for my wife, Debbie, and children Sean, Jennifer, and Laura.

Michael J. Ruckenstein

Contributors

Authored by

Michael J. Ruckenstein MD, MSc, FACS, FRCSC
Professor, Vice Chairman
Department of Otorhinolaryngology-Head and Neck Surgery
University of Pennsylvania
Philadelphia, Pennsylvania
Chapters 3, 5, 6, 7, 9, 10, 11, 14, 15

With contributions from

John J. Chi, MD
Assistant Instructor
Department of Otolaryngology-Head and Neck Surgery
University of Pennsylvania Health System
Philadelphia, Pennsylvania
Chapter 5

Marc A. Cohen, MD
Assistant Instructor
Department of Otorhinolaryngology-Head and Neck Surgery
Hospital of the University of Pennsylvania
Philadelphia, Pennsylvania
Chapter 11

Raj C. Dedhia, MD
Resident Physician
Department of Otolaryngology-Head and Neck Surgery
University of Pittsburgh Medical Center
Pittsburgh, Pennsylvania
Chapter 2

Marc D. Eisen, MD, PhD
Assistant Clinical Professor
Division of Otolaryngology (surgery)
University of Connecticut School of Medicine
Medical Director
Hartford Hospital Hearing and Balance Center
Hartford, Connecticut
Chapter 1

Elizabeth Grace, PT, MS, NCS
Director of Operations
Penn Balance Center, Penn Medicine
Neurologic Team Leader
Good Shepherd Penn Partners-Penn Therapy and Fitness
Philadelphia, Pennsylvania
Chapter 12

Jason Leibowitz, MD
Assistant Instructor
Department of Otorhinolaryngology-Head and Neck Surgery
Hospital of the University of Pennsylvania

Philadelphia, Pennsylvania
Chapter 6

Steven D. Rauch, MD
Professor
Otology and Laryngology
Harvard Medical School
Massachusetts Eye and Ear Infirmary
Boston, Massachusetts
Chapter 4

Jessica Shen, MD
Assistant Instructor
Department of Otorhinolaryngology
Hospital of University of Pennsylvania
Philadelphia, Pennsylvania
Chapter 10

Neil T. Shepard, PhD
Director, Dizziness and Balance Disorders Program
Mayo Clinic-Rochester
Professor of Audiology
Mayo Medical School
Rochester, Minnesota
Chapter 8

Jeffrey P. Staab, MD, MS
Senior Associate Consultant
Department of Psychiatry and Psychology
Mayo Clinic
Rochester, Minnesota
Chapter 13

1

Historical Perspectives

Marc D. Eisen

Introduction

Historical analysis of a disease typically follows a path from the initial description of the disease through to an accepted, mainstream understanding of the disease pathophysiology, symptomatology, and treatment. To say that Ménière's disease is "understood" would be an oversimplification, if not a falsity, and therefore its history continues to be written. This chapter highlights the early landmarks in the history of Ménière's disease, focusing on several of its aspects. The first is the description of the clinical phenomenon of what we now classify as Ménière's disease, which is credited to Prosper Ménière. Not only did Ménière astutely describe the disease, but he also anatomically localized the disease to the inner ear. The second is the identification of the temporal bone pathology associated with the disease—endolymphatic hydrops. Last is the colorful, varied, and even entertaining field of Ménière's disease treatment.

Disease Identification

Characterizing the inner ear as an organ of balance function as well as hearing function did not occur until the second half of the 19th century. Prior to that time, balance and vertigo were attributed to the central nervous system, and in fact, disorders of balance and vertigo were considered psychiatric illnesses. "Apoplectic cerebral congestion," which could be manifest as epilepsy, included unsteadiness and vertigo as part of its spectrum of symptoms. Work done in the 19th century by Flourens, however, presented good evidence that the labyrinth conferred vestibular function. He performed several lesion studies of the labyrinth in pigeons and described the vertigo and nystagmus that resulted.[1–3] Although this work convincingly demonstrated a role of the inner ear in balance and vertigo, it was not readily accepted at the time of Ménière's publications.[4]

Prosper Ménière was born in Anger on June 18, 1799.[5] He had his medical training at the Hotel Dieu in Paris, receiving his doctorate of medicine in 1828. His interests were wide and varied, from obstetrics to infectious disease to clothes and cosmetics, but his interests eventually focussed on otology.[5] He became the chief physician at the Imperial Institute for Deaf Mutes in Paris in 1838, a post he held until his death in 1862. In 1861 Ménière presented a series of papers in the *Gazette Medicale de Paris* that established the disease that bears his name.[6–9]

Two concepts were developed in these monographs. The first draws the association between the inner ear and vertigo and balance function. This association was contrary to the dogma of the day that assigned balance function and vertigo to a central nervous system locus. In order to make this association, Ménière cited the work of Flourens.[9] As another means of assigning vestibular function to the inner ear, Ménière recounts a case of a young female patient from years prior who suffered from the acute onset of hearing loss and vertigo and died days later. Ménière performed the autopsy and found an abnormal labyrinthine exudate without any neural or central nervous system disease.[10] His conclusion from this case was that the semicircular canals conferred vestibular function and when diseased could cause vertigo.[11]

The second concept was to describe a disease that included episodes of severe vertigo and frequently associated falls, but was distinct from disorders of "apoplectiform cerebral congestion" in that the pathologic site was in the inner ear rather than the brain. This distinct syndrome involved tinnitus and unilateral hearing loss in addition to the vertigo. Not only did Ménière describe the typical episodes of spinning vertigo and nausea associated with the disorder, but he also described drop attacks and the chronic low-grade disequilibrium that can persist in between episodes. Ménière also added that the tympanic membrane and middle ear were uninvolved with the disease. He explained the importance of separating this disorder from the cerebral congestion disorders, as the bloodletting and purgation commonly prescribed for cerebral congestion was not appropriate for an inner ear disorder. Ménière hoped that by defining the syndrome as a distinct entity that he would spare afflicted patients from irrational, harmful treatment instead of letting the disease run its natural course.[10] Prosper Ménière died in the year that followed publication of his seminal work. Over the course of the next few decades, the term "Ménière's disease" appeared often in otologic texts as a symptom complex involving both dizziness and auditory dysfunction. In this context, however, it was unlikely differentiated from labyrinthitis.

Several additions were made to the clinical symptomatology of Ménière's disease in the first half of the 20th century to reach our modern characterization of the disease. Crowe emphasized the characteristic fluctuations in hearing impairment.[12] The phenomenon of loudness recruitment was described by Fowler in 1937[13] and then recognized as a sequelae of Ménière's disease.[14] Aural fullness was also incorporated as a symptom.[15,16]

Histopathologic Correlate

An understanding of the pathologic entity associated with the disease did not begin to materialize until well into the 20th century. In 1928, Walter Dandy, the pioneering neurosurgeon at Johns Hopkins, reviewed a series of patients he diagnosed with Ménière's disease. He reasoned that the site of the lesion in Ménière's disease was the VIIIth nerve and not the end organ. Dandy's reached this conclusion because he could not envision a process so diffuse that it involved all three semicircular canals and the cochlea.[17] He also noted that no pathologic specimens of a Ménière's disease patient had been studied, and that the burden of proof rested on pathologic analysis, and that had yet to be described. Ironically, Samuel Crowe (an otolaryngologist) also treated and followed Dandy's patients at Johns Hopkins and ascribed Ménière's disease to a disorder of pressure or chemical changes in the endolymph.[12]

In 1938 the Bristol-based author A. J. Wright reviewed his experience with patients who presented with vertigo and hearing complaints in the absence of active middle ear pathology. Sixty-six patients were reviewed. He found one or more sites of bodily infection in all cases, which included teeth, tonsil, uterus, and maxillary sinus. Wright postulated that the pathophysiology of aural vertigo is focal bacterial labyrinthitis, based on the fact that these patients had concurrent infections.[18] At this time in the preantibiotic era, however, the prevalence of a similar finding of concurrent infection in the general population was likely substantial, and this would confound the observation. The high variability in the time course of the vertigo episodes among the patients suggests that the multiple labyrinthine diagnoses were being lumped together, including labyrinthitis, benign positional vertigo, and acoustic tumors in addition to true Ménière's disease. Nonetheless, Wright does identify the labyrinth as the site of the lesion, rather than the middle ear or eustachian tube. Neither Ménière nor Ménière's disease is mentioned in his paper.[18]

The classic description of the histopathologic correlate of Ménière's disease came in 1938 when Hallpike and Cairns reported their findings from two temporal bone specimens obtained from patients with documented disease. Both patients were treated with an VIIIth nerve section and died from surgical complications. Histopathologic analysis showed no abnormalities in the labyrinth and temporal bone except for dilatation of the saccule. They did see dilatation of endolymphatic spaces of the vestibule and cochlea with displacement of Reissner's membrane, and hence "endolymphatic hydrops." They differentiated these changes from those associated with an VIIIth nerve tumor or changes that could be due to the trauma of the intracranial surgery. The pathophysiology of such changes was postulated to be due to either excessive production of endolymph or alteration of its ionic homeostasis. One specific additional finding was that the utricle was unaltered from normal, while the saccule was dilated. They postulated that the utricle was more resistant to dilatation due to thicker walls than the saccule, and they supported their hypothesis with the finding that the utricle walls were in fact thicker than those of the saccule in normal bones. They also postulate a mechanism that can explain the paroxysmal attacks: with expansion of the endolymphatic spaces of the cochlea, the compliance of the endolymphatic system was greatly decreased, and with very small volume increases in endolymph significant pressure increases would result. With these pressure increases would come "asphyxia of the labyrinthine end-organs."[19] A corollary of their hypothesis is that acute attacks were associated with hypofunction of the affected side rather than irritation (ie, hyperfunction), as was suggested by Crowe.[12]

An apparent leap forward in the understanding of the disease came with the creation of animal models of endolymphatic hydrops by manipulating the endolymphatic sac. Hydrops in both guinea pig[20,21] and cat[22] were described and attributed to destruction of the endolymphatic sac. The association between endolymphatic sac dysfunction and Ménière's disease was strong, but yet incomplete, as endolymphatic hydrops as a histologic finding is not sufficient to explain the clinical manifestation of the disease.[23]

Treatment of Ménière's Disease

Ménière's disease has a host of seemingly insurmountable challenges to its basic study and understanding, that is, difficulty creating a complete animal model, difficulty obtaining pathological human specimens, lack of valid measurements of the disease severity and treatment efficacy, relatively low incidence and prevalence, and the natural history of the disease tending toward general improvement. Given these challenges, it is not surprising that treatments for the disease over the past century have lacked outcomes-based support. The treatments were based, rather, on honorable intent and rational thought from the physicians and researchers who brought them forth. Instead of describing the myriad individual treatments, the theories on which they were based are mentioned here.

With the histologic finding of endolymphatic hydrops, a logical target for therapeutics was to alter the fluid and electrolyte balance in the labyrinthine fluids to counteract the "vasomotor labyrinthitis" of Ménière's disease. Mygind and Dederling associated Ménière's disease with angioneurotic edema,[24] and from this concept came salt restriction. These authors also discussed the idea that altering middle ear pressure can influence endolymphatic fluid balance and alleviate the symptoms of the disease,[25] and this is the beginning of the rationale behind what has become the Meniette device. The altered endolymphatic fluid balance was attributed to osmotic pressure gradients resulting from retained endolymphatic ions.[26] Labyrinthine vasospasm was the rationale for utilizing a host of vasodilators. Most of these treatments have gone by the way of mere historical significance. Henry Williams gives an excellent account of the variety of treatments in his 1952 text.[11]

Surgical treatment for Ménière's disease shares an equally colorful past. From the time of Dandy[17,27] through most of the 20th century, severing the VIIIth nerve was described as the gold standard surgical treatment for controlling vertigo in unilateral Ménière's disease, but carried the risks associated with craniotomy. Destruction of the labyrinth had its origin when it was performed with a trephine (Houtant). Portmann used the rationale of increased endolymphatic pressure in describing an incision in the saccus endolymphaticus, propagated as endolymphatic shunt surgery.[28] Decompression of the endolymphatic chambers during episodes is the rationale for the Cody tack procedure.[29,30]

Conclusions

Our crediting of the Ménière's disease eponym to Prosper Ménière is appropriate, as Ménière not only accurately described the disease that bears his name, but he also set the pathologic site of lesion in the labyrinth. Although the identification and description of Ménière's disease as a symptom complex has remained relatively unchanged over the past century and a half, a clear understanding of the pathophysiology of the disease has been much more elusive. As a result, the literature of Ménière's disease has been rife with conjecture, empirical treatments, and uncontrolled anecdotal "evidence"—a recipe for a creative and colorful history if nothing else.

References

1. Flourens P. Recherches sur les conditions fondamentales de l'audition. *Mem Acad Roy Sci.* 1824;27 December.
2. Flourens P. Experiences sur les canaux semi-circulaires des oiseaux. *Mem Acad Roy Sci.* 1830;9:455–466.
3. Flourens P. *Recherches experimentales sure les proprietes et les fonctions du systeme nerveux dans les animaux vertebres.* Paris, France: Bailliere; 1842.
4. Ruben RJ, Harris JP. Meniere's role in the recognition of the ear as a source of vertigo: Historical perspective. In: Harris JP, ed. *Meniere's Disease.* The Hague, Netherlands: Kugler; 1999:3–13.
5. Wells WA. Dr. Prosper Meniere—historical sketch. *Laryngoscope.* 1947;57:275–293.
6. Meniere P. Congestions cerebrales apoplectiformes. *Gaz Med Paris.* 1861;16:55.
7. Meniere P. Maladies de l'oreille interne offrant les symptomes de la congestion cerebrale apoplectiforme. *Gaz Med Paris.* 1861;16:88.
8. Meniere P. Nouveaux documents relatifs aux lesions de l'oreille interne caracterisees par des symptomes de congestion cerebrale apoplectiforme. *Gaz Med Paris.* 1861;16:239.
9. Meniere P. Mémoire sur des lésions de l'oreille interne donnant lieu a des symptomes de congestion cérébrale apoplectiforme. *Gaz Med Paris.* 1861; 16:597–601.
10. Atkinson M. Meniere's original papers reprinted with an English translation together with commentaries and biographical sketch. *Acta Otolaryngol.* 1961; suppl 162:1–78.
11. Williams HL. *Meniere's disease.* Springfield, IL: Charles C Thomas; 1952.
12. Crowe SJ. Meniere's disease. *Medicine.* 1938;17:1–36.
13. Fowler EP. Measuring sensation of loudness: a new approach to the physiology of hearing and functional and differential diagnostic tests. *Arch Otolaryngol.* 1937;26:514.
14. Dix MR, Hallpike CS, Hood JD. Observations on loudness recruitment phenomenon. *J Laryngol Otol.* 1948;62:671.
15. Lindsay JR. Labyrinthine dropsy. *Laryngoscope.* 1946;56:325.
16. Cawthorne TE. Meniere's disease. *Ann Otol Rhino Laryngol.* 1947;56:18.
17. Dandy WE. Meniere's disease. Its diagnosis and a method of treatment. *Arch Surg.* 1928;16:1127–1152.
18. Wright AJ. Aural vertigo: a clinical study. *J Laryngol Otol.* 1938;53(2):97.
19. Hallpike CS, Cairns H. Observations on the pathology of Meniere's syndrome. *J Laryngol Otol.* 1938;53:625–655.
20. Kimura RS. Experimental blockage of the endolymphatic duct and sac and its effect on the inner ear of the guinea pig.

A study on endolymphatic hydrops. *Ann Otol Rhinol Laryngol.* 1967;76(3): 664–687.

21. Kimura RS, Schuknecht HF. Membranous hydrops in the inner ear of the guinea pig after obliteration of the endolymphatic sac. *Pract Oto-rhino-laryngol.* 1965;27:343.
22. Schuknecht HF, Northrop C, Igarashi M. Cochlear pathology after destruction of the endolymphatic sac in the cat. *Acta Otolaryngol.* 1968;65(5):479–487.
23. Merchant SN, Adams JC, Nadol JB, Jr. Pathophysiology of Meniere's syndrome: are symptoms caused by endolymphatic hydrops? *Otol Neurotol.* 2005; 26(1):74–81.
24. Mygind SH, Dederding D. Meniere's disease as an indicator of disturbances in the water metabolism, capillary function, and body condition. *Ann Otol Rhinol Laryngol.* 1938;47:55–62.
25. Mygind SH, Dederding D. The diagnosis and treatment of Meniere's disease. *Ann Otol Rhinol Laryngol.* 1938;47:673.
26. Furstenberg AC, Richardson G, Lathrop FD. Meniere's disease. *Arch Otolaryngol.* 1941;34:1083–1092.
27. Dandy WE. Meniere's disease: symptoms, objective findings and treatment in forty-two cases. *Arch Otolaryngol.* 1934;20(1):1–30.
28. Portmann G. The saccus endolymphaticus and an operation for draining the same for the relief of vertigo. *J Laryngol Otol.* 1927;42:809.
29. Cody DT. The tack operation for endolymphatic hydrops. *Laryngoscope.* 1969; 79(10):1737–1744.
30. Cody DT, Simonton KM, Hallberg OE. Automatic repetitive decompression of the saccule in endolymphatic hydrops (tack operation). Preliminary report. *Laryngoscope.* 1967;77(8):1480–1501.

2

Epidemiology of Ménière's Disease

Raj C. Dedhia, MD

Incidence and Prevalence

Using the Phillips' definition, incidence is the number of new cases diagnosed during a set time period (ie, 1 year) whereas prevalence is the total number of active cases.[1] The numbers for overall incidence and prevalence of Ménière's disease (MD) vary widely in the world literature. In addition to study-specific biases, the variation in diagnostic criteria for MD contributes to the inconsistency of prevalence rates between studies. The American Academy of Otolaryngology-Head and Neck Surgery (AAO-HNS) has updated its criteria twice since 1972, most recently in 1995.[2] The gradient of Ménière's disease diagnoses per AAO-HNS criteria are listed in Table 2–1. In 1988, the Japanese Society for Equilibrium Research (JSER) modified the diagnostic criteria from the Ménière's disease Research Committee of Japan proposed in 1976.[3] The 1988 criteria for definite diagnosis by JSER are listed in Table 2–2.

The 1995 criteria from AAO-HNS state that definite MD requires two or more episodes of vertigo lasting 20 minutes or longer, audiometrically documented hearing loss on at least one occasion, and tinnitus or aural fullness in the treated ear. Previous AAO-HNS criteria (endorsed in 1972) included cochlear and vestibular forms of the disease, yielding elevated prevalence rates for those studies utilizing earlier AAO-HNS criteria.

In the United States, several studies have been undertaken to assess incidence and prevalence of MD. The landmark American study was a 30-year epidemiologic study published in 1984 by Wladislavosky-Waserman et al[4] from the Mayo Clinic. Using the centralized diagnostic index maintained at the Mayo Clinic for the population of Rochester, Minnesota for the period of 1951 to 1980, the incidence was estimated at 15.3 per 100,000 per year and the prevalence 218.2 per 100,000. Of note, this study used the 1972 AAO-HNS criteria,

Table 2-1. Criteria for Diagnosis of Ménière's Disease from American Academy of Otolaryngology-Head and Neck Surgery (1995)[2]

Certain MD	Definite MD, plus histopathologic confirmation
Definite MD	1. Two or more episodes of vertigo lasting 20 minutes or longer 2. Audiometrically documented hearing loss on at least one occasion 3. Tinnitus or aural fullness in the treated ear 4. Other causes excluded
Probable MD	1. One definitive episode of vertigo 2. Audiometrically documented hearing loss on at least one occasion 3. Tinnitus or aural fullness in the treated ear 4. Other causes excluded
Possible MD	1. Episodic vertigo of the Ménière type without documented hearing loss or sensorineural hearing loss, fluctuating or fixed, with dysequilibrium but without episodes 2. Other causes excluded

Table 2-2. Criteria for Definite Diagnosis of Ménière's Disease Japanese Society for Equilibrium Research (1988)[3]

Subjective Symptoms	1. Repeated attacks of whirling vertigo 2. Fluctuating cochlear symptoms synchronized with vertiginous attack 3. No nervous symptoms except eighth nerve involvement 4. No histories that cause inner ear dysfunction such as otitis media, head injury, etc
Objective Symptoms	5. Audiometrically documented characteristic hearing loss such as low-tone hearing loss, fluctuating hearing loss, etc 6. Labyrinthine dysfunction shown by using the equilibrium test 7. Exclusion of central nervous involvement except eighth nerve based on neurologic examination 8. No clear evidence of cause of inner ear dysfunction based on neuro-otologic, physical, laboratory, and radiologic examinations

which included cochlear and vestibular forms of the disease (excluded in 1995 criteria). Celestino and Ralli[5] later applied 1995 AAO-HNS criteria to this study and yielded a lower incidence of 10.1 per 100,000.

In Europe, the countries of Finland and Italy have frequently published MD incidence and prevalence studies in the last 30 years. In 1999, Kotimaki et al[6] conducted a retrospective investigation and reported the incidence in a Finnish population to be 4.3 per 100,000 and the prevalence to be 43 per 100,000. In 2005, Havia et al[7] found a prevalence of 513 per 100,000 in southern Finland, more than 10 times the prevalence of the Kotimaki study. Although both studies used the 1995 AAO-HNS criteria, the more recent Havia study was prospective in nature, making it more robust and accurate in capturing true prevalence data. In Italy, Celestino and Ralli[5] published a study in 1991 revealing in incidence of 8.2 per 100,000 and a prevalence of 205 per 100,000. Interestingly, the authors illustrated that the availability of medical facilities influences the epidemiologic figures as there was a 3.4 times greater prevalence among hospital personnel. In the same year, Biagini et al[8] performed an incidence study of MD in Siena, Italy over a 10-year period, concluding the incidence to be 27.5 per 100,000.

In Japan, the preponderance of MD epidemiology has been carried out by Shojaku and Watanabe. In 2005, the authors conducted 15- and 25-year retrospective surveys[9] of two districts in Japan (Nishikubiki and Toyama) to evaluate incidence and prevalence of MD by 1988 JSER criteria (see Table 2–2). The average prevalence was 34.5 per 100,000 and the incidence was 5.0 per 100,000. In 1995, a sampling of another district yielded a prevalence of 17 per 100,000.[10]

Age

The age at onset of symptoms varies widely. According to the most recent literature, the peak incidence appears to occur in the seventh decade of life between the ages of 61 and 70.[7,9] Previous studies demonstrated the peak incidence to be closer to the fifth decade[5] as well as the seventh decade of life.[4] Shojaku and Watanabe demonstrated that the proportion of definite MD cases with age at onset older than 65 years increased progressively ($p>0.05$) by 5-year periods from 1980 to 2004. They posit a multifactorial theory for the forward shift of the peak incidence of MD over the last several years. In addition to elderly individuals being healthier than those of previous generations, there appears to a component of increased stress among the elderly, which may predispose patients to MD. Four of 11 patients diagnosed with MD over the age of 70 held managerial jobs in a Japanese study implying that job-related mental and physiologic stress may play a role in the etiology of MD. Additionally, today's sexa- and septuagenarians are caring for sick family members, adding to the level of mental and physical strain.[9]

Gender

Some studies delineate that males and females appear to be equally affected by MD whereas others demonstrate a predisposition toward females. The Wladislavosky-Waserman et al study at the Mayo Clinic failed to demonstrate statistical significance between genders with male incidence rate of 13.3 per 100,000 and female incidence rate of 16.3 per 100,000. Celestino and Ralli demonstrated that the incidence between men and women in the southeastern Latium region of Italy also was not statistically significant. Havia et al showed that within the population of southern Finland, women have a higher likelihood of being afflicted with MD as 13 of 1,751 women (742/100,000) and 3 of 1,350 men (222/100,000) were included in the category of definite MD. The large Japanese study carried out by Shojaku and Watanabe in 2005 illustrated that in two distinct survey populations females were significantly ($p<0.05$) predominant, 51.8% and 57.5%, respectively.

Race

With the majority of data originating from Rochester Minnesota, Italy, and Sweden, the available epidemiologic data applies primarily to Caucasians. The Japanese population also has been well-studied in the literature; prevalence and age data for Japanese patients appear to fall in the range of values from American and European studies. In 2007, the first epidemiologic study of MD in Africa was conducted in Nigeria by Ibekwe et al[11] Using retrospective data and inclusion criteria similar to 1995 AAO-HNS criteria, the prevalence was found to be 220 per 100,000, slightly higher than that of Caucasian and Japanese populations. Peak incidence in the Nigerian population was between the ages of 41 to 50. Given that the average life expectancy of native Nigerians is significantly less than that of developed countries, the peak incidence is consistent with the above-mentioned theory of aging and development of MD proposed by Shojaku and Watanabe.

Unilateral Versus Bilateral Involvement

In addition to demographic factors, nearly all epidemiology studies comment on the percentage of patients with bilateral inner ear involvement. The frequency of bilateral disease is unclear as studies report inconsistent rates ranging from 2% to 78%.[12] There appear to be two main reasons for wide range of values: lack of consensus regarding criteria for clinical diagnosis of MD and variation in length of follow-up among studies. In Japan, Kitahara[13] showed that bilateral disease was observed in 9.1% of individuals in their first year of experiencing symptoms and 41.5% of patients after 20 years of disease. This finding of a direct relationship between length of follow-up and frequency of bilateral disease has been confirmed by other authors in the literature.[14]

In 2007, House et al[12] published a study in which the primary objectives were to determine the prevalence and time interval for conversion from unilateral to bilateral involvement in MD and cochlear hydrops. Bilateral involvement was strictly defined by audiometric findings in combination with patient history of tinnitus, aural fullness, and hearing loss in the contralateral ear. In the retrospective chart review from 1959 to 2001, the authors found that MD was bilateral at presentation in 11% of patients and an additional 14% of patients converted from unilateral to bilateral MD during the follow-up period. The average time to conversion from unilateral to bilateral MD was 7.6 years.

Inheritance

Although the majority of cases of MD are sporadic, there appears to be a familial variant of MD. The familial variant represents between 5 and 15% of definite MD patients[15–17] and the pattern appears to be autosomal dominant with incomplete penetrance.[16,17] Traditionally, sporadic and familial MD are viewed as bearing a similar presentation; however, a recent study observed that familial MD had a higher association with female gender and more severe attacks compared to sporadic MD.[16] Further investigation on this topic is required.

Specific genetically acquired major histocompatibility complexes (MHC) in the form of specific human leukocyte antigens (HLA) are associated with MD patients. Several HLA types have been identified and research is ongoing to better delineate HLA associations predictive of the development of MD.

Summary

The epidemiology of Ménière's disease has been studied via clinical research for the last 50 years. Unfortunately, the definition and criteria used to characterize Ménière's disease have shifted over time, often making it difficult to compare data among studies. Additionally, a large number of the studies emanate from retrospective chart reviews, placing into question the quality of the data from the outset.

The annual incidence worldwide of Ménière's disease appears to fall between 4 per 100,000 to 28 per 100,000; alternatively, 0.004% to 0.028% of the population is newly diagnosed with MD each year. Prevalence of MD spans 17 per 100,000 to 513 per 100,000; alternatively, 0.017% to 0.513% of the population is currently afflicted with MD.

The majority of the current data reflects that the average age of onset of MD is increasing with a current peak incidence of 61 to 70 years. In Nigeria, a country in which the average 2007 life expectancy was 47 years, MD occurs earlier, with a peak incidence of 41 to 50 years. These figures corroborate the theory held by Shojaku and Watanabe that the accumulation of mental and physical stress contributes to the development of MD.

It appears that females are slightly more commonly affected by MD though some studies cite that that difference is not significant.

The Caucasian race has been well studied via Europe and the United States and the Japanese prevalence rates are comparable. There is a paucity of data related to blacks. One study from Nigeria has been carried out and revealed that prevalence rates are on the higher end of the values from the literature with roughly 0.22% of the Nigerian population carrying the diagnosis of MD.

A recent study from the House clinic helped to clarify the prevalence and development of bilateral MD. According to the results, 11% of patients have bilateral MD at diagnosis and an additional 14% develop MD with a mean elapsed time from diagnosis of 7.6 years.

The entity of MD is familial in 5% to 15% of cases with an inheritance pattern of autosomal dominance with incomplete penetrance. The genetic associations via MD-linked human leukocyte antigens have yet to be clearly delineated.

References

1. Phillips DS. *Basic Statistics for Health Science Students.* New York, NY: Freeman; 1978.
2. American Academy of Otolaryngology-Head and Neck Surgery Foundation, Committee on Hearing and Equilibrium. Guidelines for the diagnosis and evaluation of therapy in Ménière's disease. *Otolaryngol Head Neck Surg.* 1995;113(3):181–185.
3. Komatsuzaki A, Futaki T, Harada Y, et al. Ménière's disease: the guidelines for standardization of diagnostic criteria in vertiginous diseases—1987 (The Committee for Standardization of Diagnostic Criteria in Vertiginous Diseases). *Equilibrium Res.* 1988;47:247–249.
4. Wladislavosky-Waserman P, Facer GW, Mokri B, Kurland LT. Ménière's disease: a 30-year epidemiologic and clinical study in Rochester, MN, 1951–1980. *Laryngoscope.* 1984;94(8):1098–1102.
5. Celestino D, Ralli G. Incidence of Ménière's disease in Italy. *Am J Otol.* 1991;12(2):135–138.
6. Kotimaki J, Sorri M, Aantaa E, Nuutinen J. Prevalence of Ménière disease in Finland. *Laryngoscope.* 1999;109(5):748–753.
7. Havia M, Kentala E, Pyykko I. Prevalence of Ménière's disease in general population of Southern Finland. *Otolaryngol Head Neck Surg.* 2005;133(5):762–768.
8. Biagini C, Nuti D, Sensini I. Incidence of Ménière's disease in the Siena Local Health Unit 30 area. *Acta Otorhinolaryngol Ital.* 1991;11(4):379–383.
9. Shojaku H, Watanabe Y, Fujisaka M, et al. Epidemiologic characteristics of definite Ménière's disease in Japan. A long-term survey of Toyama and Niigata prefectures. *ORL J Otorhinolaryngol Relat Spec.* 2005;67(5):305–309.
10. Watanabe Y, Mizukoshi K, Shojaku H, Watanabe I, Hinoki M, Kitahara M. Epidemiological and clinical characteristics of Ménière's disease in Japan. *Acta Otolaryngol Suppl.* 1995;519:206–210.
11. Ibekwe TS, Ijaduola GT. Ménière's disease: rare or underdiagnosed among Africans. *Eur Arch Otorhinolaryngol.* 2007;264(12):1399–1403.
12. House JW, Doherty JK, Fisher LM, Derebery MJ, Berliner KI. Ménière's disease: prevalence of contralateral ear involvement. *Otol Neurotol.* 2006;27(3):355–361.
13. Kitahara M. Bilateral aspects of Ménière's disease. Ménière's disease with bilateral fluctuant hearing loss. *Acta Otolaryngol Suppl.* 1991;485:74–77.
14. Balkany TJ, Sires B, Arenberg IK. Bilateral aspects of Ménière's disease: an underestimated clinical entity. *Otolaryngol Clin North Am.* 1980;13(4):603–609.
15. Arweiler DJ, Jahnke K, Grosse-Wilde H. Ménière disease as an autosome dominant hereditary disease [in German]. *Laryngorhinootologie.* 1995;74(8):512–515.
16. Klockars T, Kentala E. Inheritance of Ménière's disease in the Finnish population. *Arch Otolaryngol Head Neck Surg.* 2007;133(1):73–77.
17. Morrison AW, Bailey ME, Morrison GA. Familial Ménière's disease: clinical and genetic aspects. *J Laryngol Otol.* 2009;123(1):29–37.

3

Pathophysiology of Ménière's Disease

Michael J. Ruckenstein

Introduction

Understanding the pathophysiology of Ménière's disease has been complicated by several factors.

Much of the dogma concerning the proposed mechanisms of inner ear dysfunction has been derived from observations of the pathology found in temporal bones of patients suffering from this disorder. Thus, the pathophysiology has been inferred from the observed pathology. However, a variety of insults to the cochlea, with noise being perhaps the best example, can lead to substantial alterations in the function of the cochlea, while resulting in no observable alterations in the structure of this organ. Thus, pathology does not always correlate with cochlear pathophysiology, and care must be taken when drawing conclusions about cochlear pathophysiology based purely on alterations in morphology.

A second obstacle to understanding the pathophysiology of Ménière's disease results from the lack of an animal model of this disorder. Animal models of endolymphatic hydrops do exist; however, these models do not replicate many of the clinical characteristics of Ménière's disease. Thus, animal research, which has provided so many insights into a variety of causes of auditory pathophysiology, offers only minimal information concerning the pathogenesis of Ménière's disease.

Data recorded from patients using electrocochleography have been used to diagnose the presence of endolymphatic hydrops and to draw conclusions concerning alterations in the physiology of the cochlea. The discussion pertaining to electrocochleography in Chapter 7, Audiometric Testing, indicates that many of these conclusions may be unfounded.

The purpose of this chapter is to provide an evidence-based review of the data currently available pertaining to the pathophysiology of Ménière's disease. It seeks to emphasize which theories are, and which are not, supported by hard data. As such, it is hoped that it will address some fundamental issues concerning current concepts of the pathogenesis of this disorder.

The Classical Model

As mentioned above, theories pertaining to the pathophysiology of Ménière's disease are based primarily on morphological observations. Thus, this discussion refers to data pertaining to cochlear pathology and their proposed relevance to cochlear pathophysiology.

The classical model of Ménière's disease evolved from early observations pertaining to cochlear fluid balance and pathology found in temporal bones of patients with Ménière's disease. In 1927, Guild proposed that the flow of endolymphatic fluid was primarily longitudinal, flowing down the length of the cochlea to be drained by the endolymphatic sac.[1] Subsequently, morphologic data derived from temporal bones of patients suffering from Ménière's disease revealed an expansion of the endolymphatic fluid compartment (the scala media) with the displacement of Reissner's membrane into the scala vestibuli.[2] Given that endolymphatic flow was felt to be longitudinal, it was hypothesized that the observed endolymphatic hydrops resulted from the obstruction of the endolymphatic drainage system at the level of the endolymphatic duct and/or sac. The presence of endolymphatic hydrops in the temporal bones of patients with Ménière's disease subsequently was confirmed by other authors, with the majority of reports indicating that it was the only consistent and significant pathology observed in this disorder.[3,4]

The identification of endolymphatic hydrops as the predominant abnormality in the labyrinthine morphology of patients with Ménière's disease led authors to speculate on how such pathology could result in the typical clinical findings associated with this disorder. The potassium (K^+) intoxication hypothesis, advanced by Lawrence and McCabe, has been the most widely accepted theory of the pathogenesis of Ménière's disease.[5] Based on observations of temporal bone pathology, Schuknecht further expanded on this theory, which can be summarized as follows:[6,7]

- Obstruction of longitudinal flow occurs at some level of the endolymphatic system. This can result from fibrosis within the ducts or swelling of the internal membranes (eg, the saccule or cochlear duct) to a point where flow is occluded.
- Pressure building up in the swollen endolymphatic system causes rupture of Reissner's membrane, allowing the mixing of endolymphatic and perilymphatic contents.
- The influx of K^+ into the perilymph causes acute dysfunction of the sensory hair cells leading to the classical symptomatology.
- Release of the built-up endolymphatic pressure permits Reissner's membrane to heal, allowing the return of normal cochlear fluid homeostatic

mechanisms and the cessation of symptoms.
- Continued cycles of membrane rupture and repair account for the episodic symptoms associated with Ménière's disease.

Analysis of the Classical Theory

The model described above seeks to explain the pathogenesis of endolymphatic hydrops and how this pathology can result in the symptoms that characterize Ménière's disease. However, although this model presents a neat and encompassing theory of pathogenesis, recent clinical and basic science data call into question many of its central tenets. As Kiang pointed out, if endolymphatic hydrops is the direct cause of the clinical manifestations of Ménière's disease, then all cases of Ménière's disease should be associated with hydrops, and all cases of hydrops should cause symptoms of Ménière's disease.[8] An important study by Rauch and colleagues did find evidence of hydrops in all temporal bones derived from patients who had suffered from Ménière's disease. However, hydrops was also found in a significant number of temporal bones derived from patients who displayed no clinical evidence of Ménière's disease.[3] The results of this study were confirmed in a subsequent study with a larger sample size.[9] These and other studies confirm that endolymphatic hydrops can frequently occur *without* symptoms of Ménière's disease.[5,10] Thus, utilizing endolymphatic hydrops and Ménière's disease synonymously to refer to a specific symptom complex associated with Ménière's disease appears to be *erroneous* and *inaccurate*.[7]

Based on temporal bone studies, Schuknecht proposed that fibrosis within the endolymphatic duct system resulted in obstruction of endolymph flow and the development of hydrops.[7] The most common site of obstruction was felt to be within the vestibular aqueduct, although other proximal sites within the duct system also could manifest fibrosis causing obstruction. However, fibrosis within the endolymphatic duct system is a fairly common finding, thus calling into question the significance of this observation. In a well-controlled study, no differences in the fibrosis in the endolymphatic system was found when temporal bone specimens derived from patients with, and without, Ménière's disease were compared.[11]

Basic scientific studies have provided further data that call into question the role of hydrops in precipitating the symptoms of Ménière's disease. As mentioned above, Guild's principle of longitudinal flow of endolymph, coupled with obstruction of this flow, was felt to play a central role in the generation of hydrops and, consequently, Ménière's disease. However, longitudinal endolymph flow has been shown to be negligible.[12,13] Regulation of endocochlear fluid volume is controlled locally, via radial flow of endolymph through the perilymph and then recycled back into the scala media via the spiral ligament and the stria vascularis.[13–15]

Although Guild's principle of longitudinal endolymphatic flow essentially has been disproved by these experiments, a considerable body of scientific literature has been dedicated to the analysis of the consequences of endolymphatic duct ligation in the animal model. Based on the temporal bone studies described above, it was felt that this might represent a good experimental model of Ménière's disease. Although most investigators now agree that this does not represent a valid model of Ménière's disease, these studies have been very instructive regarding the effects of hydrops on the cochlea.

Ligation of the endolymphatic duct can result in endolymphatic hydrops in certain animal models (eg, the guinea pig) but not in others (eg, the cat).[16] Ligation of the endolymphatic duct in the guinea pig will result in hydrops and deterioration in auditory function. However, the correlation between the progression of hydrops and auditory dysfunction is poor. Hydrops develops within days of surgery, accompanied by minimal electrophysiological evidence of cochlear dysfunction.[17] In contrast, significant deterioration in evoked potential thresholds is noted to occur for weeks to months after the degree of hydrops has stabilized. Thus, no correlation could be found between the degree of hydrops and the level of cochlear dysfunction. Furthermore, elevation in evoked potential thresholds occurred in the absence of evidence of ruptures of the labyrinthine membranes.

Animals with experimentally induced endolymphatic hydrops display many other morphological abnormalities, including cochlear hair cell loss, degeneration of the stria vascularis, and a reduction in strial Na^+, K^+-ATPase.[18,19] These changes occur during the months subsequent to the induction of hydrops, and are much more closely related with changes in cochlear function observed in these animals.[20–24] However, these findings were not found in temporal bones derived from patients with Ménière's disease.[24,25]

As described above, clinical exacerbations of Ménière's disease have been postulated to result from ruptures of Reissner's membrane after a buildup of pressure within the hydropic scala media. However, the weight of the experimental evidence is that, despite the presence of significant hydrops, there is no difference between the hydrostatic pressures recorded in the perilymph and endolymph.[21,26,27] Thus, endolymphatic expansion occurs in the absence of an increase in endolymphatic pressure, despite the fact that the magnitude of endolymph expansion typically is much greater in the experimental situation than in the human condition. Thus, the concept of endolymphatic pressure buildup leading to periodic rupture of Reissner's membrane cannot be supported by the experimental literature.

The validity of the "K^+ intoxication" hypothesis is further weakened by experimental data pertaining to electrolyte concentrations within the ducts of the hydropic cochlea. These data show that hydrops results in no change in perilymphatic or endolymphatic Na^+ and K^+ concentrations, even in the face of significant elevations in evoked potential auditory thresholds.[28]

Conclusions Regarding the Classical Model

Understanding the cochlear pathophysiology in Ménière's disease has focused on the role of hydrops in the generation of this disorder. However, recent data cast serious doubts on the role that hydrops plays in the development of the symptoms of Ménière's disease. Hydrops can be present in ears of patients who never experience symptoms of Ménière's disease. Scientific studies have failed to confirm that significant obstruction of the endolymphatic duct occurs in patients with Ménière's disease. Furthermore, endolymph flow has been shown to be radial, not longitudinal.

Animal models, although being poor representatives of Ménière's disease, have revealed considerable information concerning the effects of hydrops on the cochlea. In the animal model, hearing loss has not been found to be proportional to the degree of hydrops, but is more closely correlated with anatomic changes to the sensory and metabolic components of the cochlea. This pathology is not seen in humans with Ménière's disease. Furthermore, hydropic cochleas in animals demonstrate deterioration in function in the absence of increases in endolymphatic pressure, rupture of the labyrinthine membranes, or alterations in electrolyte content. **Thus, the clinical condition of Ménière's disease should not be equated with the pathological condition of endolymphatic hydrops.** In fact, hydrops well may not be the cause of the clinical symptomatology, but rather an **epiphenomenon** resulting from an underlying cochlear pathology.

Cochlear Pathophysiology in Ménière's Disease: New Perspectives

The study of cochlear pathophysiology as it relates to Ménière's disease has focused on the influence of hydrops on cochlear function. Yet, the significance of hydrops in the generation of the classical symptoms of Ménière's disease may well be exaggerated. If hydrops is not the primary mediator of cochlear pathology, how then can we understand the pathophysiology of this disorder? From the above discussion, it is clear that a new approach has to be taken to the understanding of Ménière's disease, one that includes, but does not focus on, the role of hydrops. At present, it is reasonable to conclude that very little actually is known about the underlying pathophysiology of Ménière's disease. The following discussion represents a somewhat speculative attempt at explaining the manifestations of Ménière's disease, based on what is known about different pathophysiologic mechanisms of cochlear dysfunction. It is by no means meant to be a definitive explanation of the disorder, but rather a vehicle to facilitate the consideration of alternate mechanisms of inner ear dysfunction in Ménière's disease, based on currently accepted scientific data.

Are There Analogies to be Drawn Between Ménière's Disease and Other Inner Ear Pathologies?

A hallmark of this disorder is an "active" period of disease, characterized by episodic vertigo, fluctuations in hearing, and episodic exacerbations of tinnitus. With time, the disorder tends to stabilize, leaving a permanent dysfunction of the inner ear, manifesting as hearing loss, chronic tinnitus, and imbalance. Thus, any explanation of the symptoms of Ménière's disease must incorporate a disease process that can cause a reversible cochleovestibular dysfunction, leading to a permanent cochleovestibular loss.

Several inner ear disorders can manifest this pattern, including acoustic trauma, ototoxicity, and certain genetic forms of hearing loss. Noise can exert both temporary (TTS) and permanent

(PTS) threshold shifts. Particularly relevant to this discussion is the fact that noise can induce a substantial TTS that manifests no morphologic abnormalities.[29] Only when the loss becomes irreversible (PTS) do morphologic abnormalities appear. Similarly, ototoxins, most notably salicylates, can induce significant reversible cochlear dysfunction in the absence of abnormalities in cochlear morphology.[30] Other examples of potentially reversible forms of hearing loss include viral infections and other immune-mediated inner ear diseases.[31] Acoustic neuromas, when small, also can manifest hearing loss that may fluctuate in response to steroid administration.[32] Fluctuations are also noted to occur during the progressive hearing losses attributed to genetic etiologies.[33]

These examples are not cited to suggest that they may result in Ménière's disease. Rather, they are discussed to implicate a possible final common pathway that could mediate the fluctuations in cochleovestibular function seen in Ménière's disease. Perhaps some analogies can be drawn between known pathophysiologic mechanisms of hearing loss and Ménière's disease.

Genetics of Ménière's Disease

In the last decade, tremendous advances have been made in the application of molecular biologic techniques to the study of genetic hearing loss and other forms of inner ear disease. It is likely that one day, the application of these techniques will lead to the discovery of the underlying pathophysiology of Ménière's disease. Based on our current level of knowledge, can we speculate about potential genetic abnormalities that may result in Ménière's disease?

As noted above, genetic forms of hearing loss may result in fluctuating, progressive hearing loss.[33] However, the vast majority of cases of Ménière's disease are sporadic, with only approximately 5% of cases demonstrating a familial pattern.[34] In cases of familial Ménière's disease, an autosomal dominant pattern of inheritance with reduced penetrance is most commonly observed.[34,35] In some studies, familial Ménière's disease has been strongly associated with a family history of migraines[36,37] The possibility that a common pathology links Ménière's disease and migraines is intriguing. Nonetheless, the majority of cases of Ménière's disease are sporadic and are not associated with a personal or family history of migraines.[39]

The COCH gene mutation associated with DFNA9 is associated with hearing loss and vertigo and received some attention as a potential gene coding for Ménière's disease. However, patients with Ménière's disease do not manifest COCH mutatons.[39] Possible linkage to chromosome 14 was noted in one study of families and to chromosome 12p12.3 in another.[40,41] Thus, we are still far from finding a gene that codes for a familial form of Ménière's disease. Identifying such a gene and it's function would be as tremendous advance in the study of Ménière's disease as it would point to site of lesion that could result in the observed pathology.

Inner Ear Channels and Conductances as Possible Lesion Sites

There are many examples of neuropathology resulting from abnormal function of cellular channels and conductances. The inner ear is replete with a wide variety of channels and conductances, some of which appear to be unique to the inner ear. A relatively recent paper hypothesized that Ménière's disease may result from a channelopathy.[42] The author notes to the following factors that point to the possibility that Ménière's disease is a channelopathy.

- The presence of endolymphatic hydrops possibly indicates an abnormality in fluid and electrolyte balance that could result from dysfunction in one or more labyrinthine electrolyte channels
- Mutations in genes that code for ion channels result in hereditary deafness
- Anticipation is observed in familial Ménière's disease and other neurologic disorders that are caused by channelopathies
- Many patients with channelopathies are responsive to acetazolamide, a drug that has also proven effective in Ménière's disease

Unfortunately, numerous problems are associated with the channelopathy hypothesis. Patients with Ménière's disease typically do not manifest any other associated pathologies, so the channel affected would have to be unique to the inner ear. Acetazolamide does not appear to have any specific therapeutic benefits for patients with Ménière's disease, beyond those that can be attributed to a placebo effect (see Medical Treatment, Chapter 10). Thus far, no genetic mutations associated with Ménière's disease have been identified. In addition, anticipation may, or may not, be a finding in patients with familial forms of Ménière's disease.[34] Nonetheless, a inherited or acquired defect in one or more unique labyrinthine ion channels remains an intriguing avenue of research.

Noise-Induced Hearing Loss: Are There Analogies to Ménière's Disease?

Noise-induced TTS causes a flaccidity of hair cell stereocilia, the recovery from which is dependent on the cell's ability to generate and utilize energy stored in the form of adenosine triphosphate (ATP).[29,43] Free radical formation is a major mediator of acoustic trauma, which directly affects cells of the organ of Corti and stria vascularis.[44] Decreased cochlear blood flow (secondary to free radical formation), increased intracellular calcium concentrations, and glutamate ototoxicity also play roles in mediating acoustic trauma.[44] Endogenous defense against free radical damage is likely mediated by glutathione.[45] It would be attractive to hypothesize that a progressive, degenerative inner ear disorder manifesting fluctuations in inner ear function could be due to a defect in the glutathione cytoprotective pathway. The inner ear would be less able to respond to routine challenges, initially manifesting a temporary abnormality (analogous to a TTS) and then ultimately succumbing to permanent dysfunction (analogous to a PTS). The problem with this hypothesis is that all pathologies mediated by free radicals, including noise and ototoxin exposure, result in morphological changes including loss of hair cells and cells of the stria vascularis and spiral ligament. As noted above, such pathology is not seen in temporal bones derived from patients with Ménière's disease.

Other Symptoms Associated with Ménière's Disease

Aural Fullness

The plugged sensation associated with acute exacerbations of Ménière's disease is an intriguing symptom that has not been adequately explained. Clinicians often relate to their patients that this represents a swelling of the hydropic labyrinthine membranes. Although this may be a satisfying explanation from the patient's point of view, it is untenable from a scientific perspective. Even if clinical exacerbations of Ménière's disease were caused by acute hydrops, which they do not appear to be, the inner ear is not a sensate structure, and could not convey this information to the brain. The minute volume of endolymph that accumulates in hydrops could hardly distend the round window membrane sufficiently to mimic the sensation caused by otitis media.

An alternative explanation for the sensation of aural fullness can be provided. The middle ear transfer function dictates that conductive hearing loss primarily affects the lower frequencies of hearing. From a young age, humans learn to associate low-frequency hearing loss with middle ear pathologies that also cause aural fullness (eg, otitis media). Exacerbations of Ménière's disease typically are associated with an acute deterioration of hearing in the low frequencies, which are the same frequencies affected by a conductive hearing loss. Therefore, it would seem reasonable to conclude that Ménière's disease evokes a sensation of aural fullness based on prior learned associations. A similar phenomenon is seen in patients with conductive hearing loss secondary to otosclerosis. These patients often complain of a sensation of aural fullness, despite the fact that they display normal middle ear aeration.

Loudness Intolerance

Loudness intolerance (hypercusis) is a frequent complaint in patients with Ménière's disease, as it is in any patient suffering form cochlear pathology involving the outer hair cells. It is the outer hair cells that confer on the basilar membrane its exquisite fine tuning properties. Under normal conditions, each region of the basilar membrane is finely tuned to a specific frequency. Thus, a stimulus of any particular frequency will elicit a response in only a certain number of neurons. Pathology that interferes with OHC function results in a loss of these fine-tuning properties. Hair cells, and thus neurons, become broadly tuned, and will respond to a broader range of stimulus frequencies. Because of these broad tuning characteristics, a suprathreshold stimulus will excite a larger population of neurons in the pathological cochlea than it would under normal conditions.[46–48] Because the number of afferent fibers activated is one mechanism by which stimulus intensity is coded, patients with Ménière's disease, as well as with other cochlear pathologies, will perceive sound stimuli as being uncomfortably loud.

Binaural Diplacusis

Altered pitch perception in the affected ear is another symptom associated with Ménière's disease. Like recruitment, this symptom can be attributed to an alteration in basilar membrane tuning properties. In the abnormal ear, neurons respond to a broader range of stimulus frequencies. However, due to central nervous system preconditioning, the brain interprets any activity in a particular neuron as resulting from a stimulus of its normal, characteristic frequency. Thus, a single stimulus, simultaneously processed by the normal and abnormal cochlea, will be perceived as two different stimuli by the CNS. Binaural diplacusis is particularly notable in patients with Ménière's disease due to two factors. Ménière's disease is one of the few forms of cochlear pathology that is characterized by asymmetry. In contrast to symmetric pathologies, such as presbycusis or noise-induced hearing loss, patients with Ménière's disease will possess ears with different tuning properties. In addition, pathology in Ménière's disease typically affects the "speech frequency" region of the cochlea. Thus, patients with Ménière's disease will be confronted by multiple sound stimuli that elicit binaural diplacusis.

Role of the Central Nervous System

One of the most fascinating aspects of Ménière's disease is that this peripheral inner ear disorder exhibits a substantial modulation by the CNS. It has been well documented that the incidence of acute exacerbations of the disorder can be significantly reduced by the institution of nonspecific or placebo treatments.[49,50] Such nonspecific effects are substantial, demonstrating a significant reduction in vertiginous episodes in 60% to 80% of patients. Discussions within the clinical literature all too frequently have focused on whether small differences between so-called specific and nonspecific therapies are significant. Such discussions obscure the critical observation that the substantial nonspecific effects of treatment are frequently of much greater magnitude than the minimal extra benefit conferred by the "specific" treatment.

There are three mechanisms by which the CNS can influence the cochlea. The efferent neurons, which descend to the cochlea via the crossed and uncrossed olivocochlear tracts, synapse primarily on the outer hair cells. Activation of the efferent pathways inhibits outer hair cell function, diminishing the fine tuning properties and broadening basilar membrane tuning.[51] The autonomic nervous system primarily influences tone of the vascular beds feeding the cochlea. Lastly, the neuroendocrine system may affect the cochlea in an, as yet, undetermined fashion. Presumably, this system may modulate cochlear metabolic function as steroid receptors do exist in the cochlea, primarily within the stria vascularis.[52,53] Currently, there are no scientific data to determine which of these systems may be involved in Ménière's disease. We can speculate that the efferent system might be involved in acute attacks, as broadened cochlear tuning is certainly evident during clinical exacerbations. Similarly, alterations in autonomic activity might adversely affect cochlear metabolic activity by modifying vascular tone, thus precipitating an acute exacerbation. Chronic aberrations in autonomic control could lead to permanent pathologic changes in the cochlea. The neuroendocrine system typically exerts chronic modulating effects on target organs, as opposed to mediating acute changes in function.

Thus, it would likely have a more subtle role to play in Ménière's disease than the other two control systems. It is clear that research is required in this area, as understanding the mechanisms by which the CNS can exert an effect on Ménière's disease may be the key to developing an effective treatment for this disorder.

Conclusions

This chapter explored the current status of our understanding of the pathophysiology of cochlear dysfunction in Ménière's disease. It emphasized that the classical model in which hydrops mediates cochlear pathophysiology cannot be supported by current scientific data. New approaches to the understanding of Ménière's disease are required if this disease process is ever to be understood and effectively treated. Based on current scientific knowledge, some examples of alternative explanations for the etiology and pathogenesis of the symptoms associated with Ménière's disease were provided. These explanations are not meant to be definitive or exhaustive. Rather, they are meant to orient thought and discussion concerning the pathogenesis of Ménière's disease in a new, and hopefully productive, direction.

References

1. Guild SR. The circulation of the endolymph. *Am J Anat.* 1927;39:57–81.
2. Hallpike CS, Cairns H. Observations on the pathology of Ménière's syndrome. *J Laryngol Otol.* 1938;53:625–655.
3. Rauch SD, Merchant SN, Thedinger BA. Ménière's syndrome and endolymphatic hydrops. Double-blind temporal bone study. *Ann Otol Rhinol Laryngol.* 1989;98(11):873–883.
4. Merchant SN, Adams JC, Nadol JB, Jr. Pathophysiology of Ménière's syndrome: are symptoms caused by endolymphatic hydrops? *Otol Neurotol.* 2005; 26(1):74–81.
5. Lawrence M, McCabe BF. Inner-ear mechanics and deafness. Special consideration of Ménière's syndrome. *J Am Med Assoc.* 1959;171:1927–1932.
6. Schuknecht HF, Benitez JT, Beekhuts J. Further observations on the pathology of Ménière's disease. *Ann Otol Rhinol Laryngol.* 1962;71:1039–1053.
7. Schuknecht HF, Ruther A. Blockage of longitudinal flow in endolymphatic hydrops. *Eur Arch Otorhinolaryngol.* 1991; 248(4):209–217.
8. Kiang NYS. An auditory physiologist's view of Ménière's syndrome. In: Nadol JB, Jr, ed. *Second International Symposium on Ménière's disease.* Amsterdam/Milano: Kugler & Ghedini; 1989:427–432.
9. Merchant SN, Rauch SD, Nadol JBJr. Ménière's disease. [Review] [142 refs]. *Eur Arch Otorhinolaryngol.* 1995;252(2): 63–75.
10. Vasama JP, Linthicum FH,Jr. Ménière's disease and endolymphatic hydrops without Ménière's symptoms: temporal bone histopathology. *Acta Otolaryngol (Stockh).* 1999;119(3):297–301.
11. Wackym PA, Linthicum FH Jr, Ward PH, House WF, Micevych PE, Bagger-Sjoback D. Re-evaluation of the role of the human endolymphatic sac in Ménière's disease. *Otolaryngol Head Neck Surg.* 1990;102(6):732–744.
12. Salt AN, Thalmann R, Marcus DC, Bohne BA. Direct measurement of longitudinal endolymph flow rate in the guinea pig cochlea. *Hear Res.* 1986;23(2):141–151.
13. Salt AN. Regulation of endolymphatic fluid volume [Review] [18 refs]. *Ann N Y Acad Sci.* 2001;942:306–312.
14. Salt AN, Ohyama K, Thalmann R. Radial communication between the perilym-

phatic scalae of the cochlea. I: Estimation by tracer perfusion. *Hear Res.* 1991; 56(1–2):29–36.
15. Salt AN, Ohyama K, Thalmann R. Radial communication between the perilymphatic scalae of the cochlea. II: Estimation by bolus injection of tracer into the sealed cochlea. *Hear Res.* 1991;56(1–2): 37–43.
16. Kimura RS. Animal models of endolymphatic hydrops. *Am J Otolaryngol.* 1982;3(6):447–451.
17. Salt AN, DeMott J. Time course of endolymph volume increase in experimental hydrops measured in vivo with an ionic volume marker. *Hear Res.* 1994; 74(1–2):165–172.
18. Kimura RS. Animal models of endolymphatic hydrops. *Am J Otolaryngol.* 1982;3(6):447–451.
19. Ichimiya I, Adams JC, Kimura RS. Changes in immunostaining of cochleas with experimentally induced endolymphatic hydrops. *Ann Otol Rhinol Laryngol.* 1994;103(6):457–468.
20. Horner KC. Review: morphological changes associated with endolymphatic hydrops. *Scanning Microsc.* 1993;7(1): 223–238.
21. Horner KC. Functional changes associated with experimentally induced endolymphatic hydrops. *Hear Res.* 1993;68(1):1–18.
22. Horner KC, Guilhaume A. Ultrastructural changes in the hydropic cochlea of the guinea-pig. *Eur J Neurosci.* 1995;7(6): 1305–1312.
23. Horner KC. Auditory and vestibular function in experimental hydrops. *Otolaryngol Head Neck Surg.* 1995;112(1): 84–89.
24. Nadol JB Jr, Thornton AR. Ultrastructural findings in a case of Ménière's disease. *Ann Otol Rhinol Laryngol.* 1987; 96(4):449–454.
25. Keithley EM, Horowitz S, Ruckenstein MJ. Na, K-ATPase in the cochlear lateral wall of human temporal bones with endolymphatic hydrops. *Ann Otol Rhinol Laryngol.* 1995;104(11):858–863.
26. Takeuchi S, Takeda T, Saito H. Pressure relationship between perilymph and endolymph in guinea pigs. *Acta Otolaryngol.* 1990;109(1–2):93–100.
27. Takeuchi S, Takeda T, Saito H. Pressure relationship between perilymph and endolymph associated with endolymphatic infusion. *Ann Otol Rhinol Laryngol.* 1991;100(3):244–248.
28. Sziklai I, Ferrary E, Horner KC, Sterkers O, Amiel C. Time-related alteration of endolymph composition in an experimental model of endolymphatic hydrops. *Laryngoscope.* 1992;102(4):431–438.
29. Saunders JC, Cohen YE, Szymko YM. The structural and functional consequences of acoustic injury in the cochlea and peripheral auditory system: a five year update. *J Acoust Soc Am.* 1991; 90(1):136–146.
30. Jung TT, Rhee CK, Lee CS, Park YS, Choi DC. Ototoxicity of salicylate, nonsteroidal antiinflammatory drugs, and quinine. *Otolaryngol Clin North Am.* 1993;26(5):791–810.
31. Ruckenstein MJ. Autoimmune inner ear disease. *Curr Opin Otolaryngol Head Neck Surg.* 2004;12(5):426–430.
32. Aronzon A, Ruckenstein MJ, Bigelow DC. The efficacy of corticosteroids in restoring hearing in patients undergoing conservative management of acoustic neuromas. *Otol Neurotol.* 2003;24(3): 465–468.
33. Brookhouser PE, Worthington DW, Kelly WJ. Fluctuating and/or progressive sensorineural hearing loss in children. *Laryngoscope.* 1994;104(8 pt 1):958–964.
34. Morrison AW, Bailey ME, Morrison GA. Familial Ménière's disease: clinical and genetic aspects. *J Laryngol Otol.* 2009;123(1):29–37.
35. Frykholm C, Larsen HC, Dahl N, Klar J, Rask-Andersen H, Friberg U. Familial Ménière's disease in five generations. *Otol Neurotol.* 2006;27(5):681–686.

36. Cha YH, Kane MJ, Baloh RW. Familial clustering of migraine, episodic vertigo, and Ménière's disease. *Otol Neurotol.* 2008;29(1):93–96.
37. Jen JC. Recent advances in the genetics of recurrent vertigo and vestibulopathy. *Curr Opin Neurol.* 2008;21(1):3–7.
38. Rassekh CH, Harker LA. The prevalence of migraine in Ménière's disease. *Laryngoscope.* 1992;102(2):135–138.
39. Sanchez E, Lopez-Escamez JA, Lopez-Nevot MA, Lopez-Nevot A, Cortes R, Martin J. Absence of COCH mutations in patients with Ménière disease. *Eur J Hum Genet.* 2004;12(1):75–78.
40. Morrison AW, Johnson KJ. Genetics (molecular biology) and Ménière's disease. *Otolaryngol Clin North Am.* 2002; 35(3):497–516.
41. Klar J, Frykholm C, Friberg U, Dahl N. A Ménière's disease gene linked to chromosome 12p12.3. *Am J Med Genet B Neuropsychiatr Genet.* 2006;141B(5): 463–467.
42. Gates P. Hypothesis: could Ménière's disease be a channelopathy? [Review] [20 refs]. *Intern Med J.* 2005 Aug;35(8): 488–489.
43. Canlon B. The effect of acoustic trauma on the tectorial membrane, stereocilia, and hearing sensitivity: possible mechanisms underlying damage, recovery, and protection. *Scand Audiol Suppl.* 1988;27:1–45.
44. Le Prell CG, Yamashita D, Minami SB, Yamasoba T, Miller JM. Mechanisms of noise-induced hearing loss indicate multiple methods of prevention. *Hear Res.* 2007;226(1–2):22–43.
45. Usami S, Hjelle OP, Ottersen OP. Differential cellular distribution of glutathione—an endogenous antioxidant—in the guinea pig inner ear. *Brain Res.* 1996;743(1–2):337–340.
46. Evans EF, Palmer AR. Proceedings: Responses of units in the cochlear nerve and nucleus of the cat to signals in the presence of bandstop noise. *J Physiol.* 1975;252(2):60P–62P.
47. Evans EF, Wilson JP. Cochlear tuning properties: concurrent basilar membrane and single nerve fiber measurements. *Science.* 1975;190(4220):1218–1221.
48. Evans EF. The frequency response and other properties of single fibres in the guinea-pig cochlear nerve. *J Physiol.* 1972;226(1):263–287.
49. Torok N. Old and new in Ménière disease. *Laryngoscope.* 1977;87(11):1870–1877.
50. Ruckenstein MJ, Rutka JA, Hawke M. The treatment of Ménière's disease: Torok revisited. *Laryngoscope.* 1991; 101(2):211–218.
51. Cooper NP, Guinan JJ Jr. Efferent-mediated control of basilar membrane motion. *J Physiol.* 2006;576(pt 1):49–54.
52. Rarey KE, Lohuis PJ, ten Cate WJ. Response of the stria vascularis to corticosteroids. *Laryngoscope.* 1991;101(10): 1081–1084.
53. Pitovski DZ, Drescher MJ, Drescher DG. Glucocorticoid receptors in the mammalian inner ear: RU 28362 binding sites. *Hear Res.* 1994;77(1–2):216–220.

4

Histopathology

Steven D. Rauch, MD

Introduction

Although the essential histopathologic feature of Ménière's disease, idiopathic endolymphatic hydrops, was described in 1938, new findings continue to emerge. A detailed appreciation for the histopathology of Ménière's disease is essential to deepening our understanding of the pathophysiology and clinical features of the condition.

Endolymphatic Hydrops

In 1938, Hallpike and Cairns[1] in England, and Yamakawa[2] in Japan, independently reported the histopathologic finding of endolymphatic hydrops in temporal bones from patient with Ménière's disease. Numerous subsequent reports confirmed these findings.[3–16] Temporal bone studies by Rauch et al[17] and by Merchant et al[18] showed that nearly all patients with clinical Ménière's disease in life exhibit cochleosaccular endolymphatic hydrops post mortem (Fig 4–1). Although cochleosaccular hydrops is the predominant histopathologic change observed in Ménière temporal bones, there is wide variability in the severity of these hydropic changes and there may be hydropic distention of the utricle and/or semicircular canal ampullae. The hydrops is idiopathic, with no other apparent temporal bone pathology that might cause it. This distinguishes the hydrops of Ménière's disease from that seen in other conditions, such as Mondini dysplasia, trauma, labyrinthitis, or syphilis. The hydropic distention of the cochlea and labyrinth sometimes causes thinning, outpouching, and ruptures. Distortion and collapse of the walls of the ampullae, utricle, and cochlear duct can be observed in severe cases. It is important to note that endolymphatic hydrops is not synonymous with Ménière's disease. There are many instances of postmortem temporal

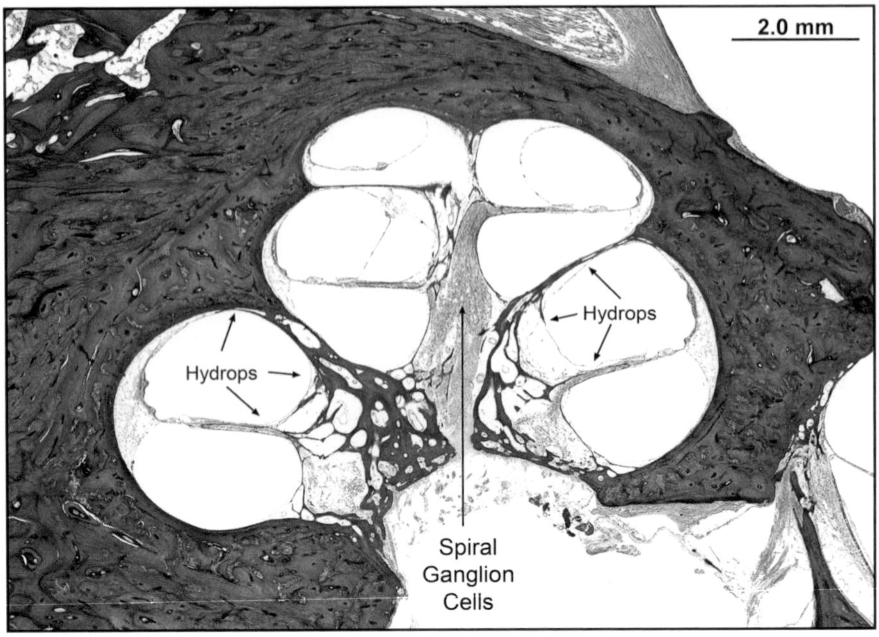

A

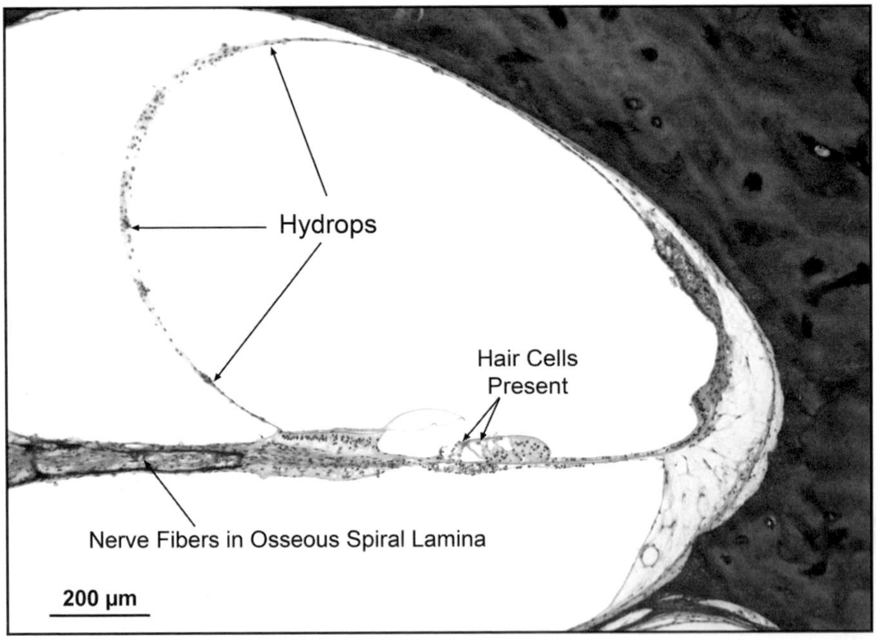

B

Fig 4–1. Idiopathic endolymphatic hydrops in Ménière's disease. **A.** Low magnification histopathologic mid-modiolar section of the inner ear of a patient with classic Ménière's disease. Endolymphatic spaces are markedly distended. Spiral ganglioin cell population is largely intact. **B.** High magnification of upper middle turn of the same cochlea. Note preservation of hair cells. Sections are embedded in celloidin, sectioned at 20 μm thickness, and stained with hematoxylin and eosin. Courtesy of Saumil N. Merchant, MD, Massachusetts Eye and Ear Infirmary, Boston.

bones with idiopathic endolymphatic hydrops from patients who never exhibited clinical symptoms of Ménière's disease (Fig 4–2).

Vestibular Fibrosis

Fibrous tissue proliferating within the vestibule in Ménière's disease is a common observation. Fibrous bands may bridge between the utricular macula and the undersurface of the stapes footplate. Nadol[19] has speculated that this may account for the positive Hennebert's sign (positive "fistula test" without a fistula) seen in approximately 30% of Ménière ears.

Sensory Lesions

In the majority of Ménière cases reported, light microscopy of temporal bone sections shows sensory hair cells of the cochlea[16] and labyrinth[20] to be substantially intact. A quantitative analysis of vestibular hair cells using higher resolution Nomarski optics has shown a specific loss of type II vestibular hair

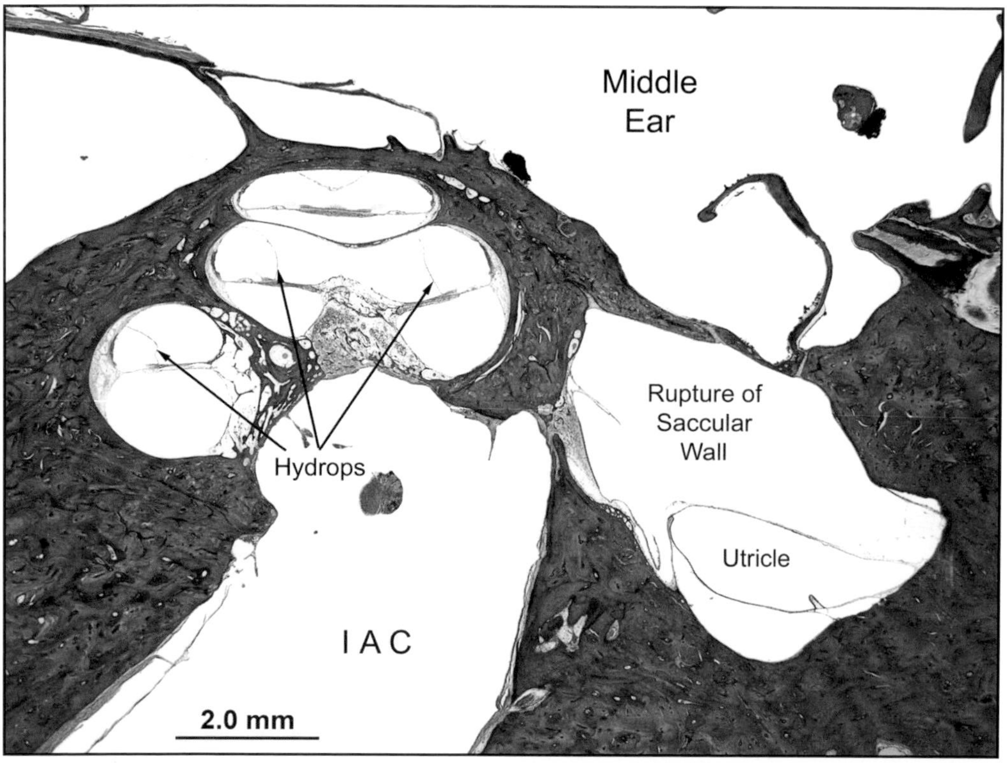

Fig 4–2. Idiopathic endolymphatic hydrops without Ménière's disease. This low magnification mid-modiolar section of the cochlea and vestibule exhibits cochleosaccular endolymphatic hydrops indistinguishable from Ménière's disease. However, this patient never suffered any vertigo. Section embedded in celloidin, sectioned at 20 µm thickness, and stained with hematoxylin and eosin. Courtesy of Saumil N. Merchant, MD, Massachusetts Eye and Ear Infirmary, Boston.

cells from all three semicircular canal cristae, and both utricular and saccular maculae in Ménière ears compared to age-matched controls.[21] In advanced disease, more extensive morphologic changes, including loss of cochlear hair cells, atrophy of supporting cells in the organ of Corti, distortion and atrophy of the tectorial membrane, and atrophy of the cristae, have been observed.[22] Most electron microscopic studies of Ménière temporal bones have failed to show changes of the inner ear, cochlear nerve, or vestibular nerve, but Kimura et al[23] and Nadol and Thornton[24] showed significant pathology in surviving cochlear hair cells, including fusion of stereocilia, disruption of cuticular bodies, and basalward displacement of some outer hair cells with loss of contact with the cuticular plate.

Neural Lesions

Neuronal cell counts of the spiral ganglion[16] and Scarpa's ganglion[20] have been reported to be normal. However, the higher resolution quantitative study by Tsuji et al[21] showed a reduction of Scarpa's ganglion cells in Ménière ears compared to age-matched normals. There is an isolated loss of neurons from the cochlear apex seen in approximately 10% of Ménière temporal bones. There also may be some loss of nerve fibers in the osseous spiral lamina.[25] Nadol and Thornton[24] compared the affected to the unaffected side of unilateral Ménière's disease at the ultrastructural level. They observed a striking and statistically significant reduction in the number of afferent nerve endings and afferent synapses at the base of both inner and other cochlear hair cells on the affected side.

Endolymphatic Sac and Vestibular Aqueduct

Hallpike and Cairns[1] described a decrease in the amount of "loose" connective tissue surrounding the endolymphatic sac in Ménière's disease, though noting that this finding was also seen in some normal temporal bones. A variety of pathologic changes in the endolymphatic sac have been described since then, including hypoplasia of the vestibular aqueduct,[26–28] hypoplasia of the endolymphatic sac,[26] decreased vascularization of the sac,[29] and perisaccular fibrosis.[30] However, others studies have challenged these findings.[31–34]

Summary

Since Hallpike and Cairns, and Yamakawa, originally described the temporal bone histopathology of Ménière's disease in 1938, we have learned that it is characterized by idiopathic cochleosaccular endolymphatic hydrops, often with involvement of the ampullae and utricle. There is preferential degeneration of type II vestibular hair cells and ganglion cells of Scarpa's ganglion. Ultrastructurally, there is deafferentation of cochlear hair cells. Some hair cells show distortion of their stereocilia and cuticular plate. There are conflicting opinions about morphologic abnormalities or changes of the endolymphatic sac.

References

1. Hallpike CS, Cairns H. Observations on the pathology of Ménière's syndrome. *J Laryngol Otol.* 1938;53:625–655.
2. Yamakawa K. Über die pathologische Veränderung bei einem Ménière-

Kranken. *J Otorhinolaryngol Soc Jpn.* 1938;4:2310–2312.
3. Altmann F, Fowler EP Jr. Histological findings in Ménière's symptom complex. *Ann Otol Rhinol Laryngol.* 1943;52: 52–80.
4. Altmann F, Kornfeld M. Histological studies of Ménière's disease. *Ann Otol Rhinol Laryngol.* 1965;74:915–943.
5. Cawthorne T. Ménière's disease. *Ann Otol Rhinol Laryngol.* 1947;56:18–38.
6. Day KM, Lindsay JR. Hydrops of the labyrinth. Case report: coagulation operation, clinical course and histopathology. *Laryngoscope.* 1949;59:213–227.
7. Hallpike CS, Harrison MS. Ménière's disease treated by Portmann's operation: report and clinicopathological study of a case. *Arch Otolaryngol.* 1954;60:141–144.
8. Kristensen HK. Histopathology in Ménière's disease. *Acta Otolaryngol (Stockh).* 1961;53:237–248.
9. Lawrence M, McCabe BF. Inner ear mechanics and deafness: special consideration of Ménière's syndrome. *JAMA.* 1959;171:1927–1932.
10. Lindsay JR. Labyrinthine dropsy and Ménière's disease. *Arch Otolaryngol.* 1942;35:853–867.
11. Lindsay JR. Ménière's disease: histopathologic observations. *Arch Otolaryngol.* 1944;39:313–318.
12. Lindsay JR. Labyrinthine dropsy. *Laryngoscope.* 1946;56:325–341.
13. Lindsay JR, Schulthess GV. An unusual case of labyrinthine hydrops. *Acta Otolaryngol (Stockh).* 1958;49:315–324.
14. Nager FR. Zur Histopathologie des Ohrschwwindels. *Pract Otorhinolaryngol.* 1949;11:360–377.
15. Rollin J. Zur Kenntnis des Labyrinthhydrops und des durch ihn bedingten Ménière. *HNO.* 1940;331:73–109.
16. Schuknecht HF, Benitez JT, Beekhuis J. Further observations on the pathology of Ménière's disease. *Ann Otol Rhinol Laryngol.* 1962;71:1039–1053.
17. Rauch SD, Merchant SN, Thedinger BA. Ménière's syndrome and endolymphatic hydrops: a double-blind temporal bone study. *Ann Otol Rhinol Laryngol.* 1989; 98:873–883.
18. Merchant SN, Adams JC, Nadol JB Jr. Pathophysiology of Ménière's disease: are the symptoms caused by endolymphatic hydrops? *Otol Neurotol.* 2005;26: 74–81.
19. Nadol JB Jr. Positive Hennebert's sign in Ménière's disease. *Arch Otolaryngol.* 1977;103:524–530.
20. Richter E. Quantitative study of Scarpa's ganglion and vestibular sense organs in endolymphatic hydrops. *Ann Otol Rhino Laryngol.* 1981;90:121–125.
21. Tsuji K, Velazquez-Villasenor L, Rauch SD, Glynn RJ, Wall C, Merchant SN. Temporal bone studies of the human peripheral vestibular system: 4. Ménière's disease. *Ann Otol Rhinol Laryngol.* 2000; 109(pt 2, suppl 181):26–31.
22. Schuknecht HF. Ménière's disease. In: English GM, ed. *Otolaryngology.* Philadelphia, PA: Lippincott; 1989:1–23.
23. Kimura RS, Ota CY, Schuknecht HF, Takahashi T. Electron microscopic observations in bilateral Ménière's disease. *Ann Otol Rhinol Laryngol.* 1976;85:791–801.
24. Nadol JB, Thornton AR. Ultrastructural findings in a case of Ménière's disease. *Ann Otol Rhinol Laryngol.* 1987;96:449–454.
25. Spoendlin H, Balle V, Bock G, et al. Multicentre evaluation of the temporal bones obtained from a patient with suspected Ménière's disease. *Acta Otolaryngol (Stockh).* 1992;499:1–21.
26. Hebbar GK, Rask-Anderson H, Linthicum FH. Three-dimensional analysis of 61 human endolymphatic ducts and sacs in ears with and without Ménière's disease. *Ann Otol Rhinol Laryngol.* 1991; 100:219–225.
27. Rizvi SS, Smith LE. Idiopathic endolymphatic hydrops and the vestibular aqueduct. *Ann Otol Rhinol Laryngol.* 1981;90:77–79.
28. Sando I, Ikeda M. The vestibular aqueduct in patients with Ménière's disease. A temporal bone histopathological investigation. *Acta Otolaryngol (Stockh).* 1984;97:558–570.

29. Ikeda M, Sando I. Vascularity of endolymphatic sac in Ménière's disease. A histopathologic study. *Ann Otol Rhinol Laryngol.* 1985;94(suppl 118):6–10.
30. Ikeda M, Sando I. Endolymphatic duct and sac in patients with Ménière's disease. A temporal bone histopathologic study. *Ann Otol Rhinol Laryngol.* 1984; 93:540–546.
31. Fraysse BG, Alonso A, House WF. Ménière's disease and endolymphatic hydrops. Clinical-histopathological correlations. *Ann Otol Rhinol Laryngol.* 1980;89(suppl 76):2–22.
32. Platenga KF, Browning GG. The vestibular aqueduct and endolymphatic sac and duct in endolyphatic hydrops. *Arch Otolaryngol.* 1979;105:546–552.
33. Wackym PA, Linthicum FH, Ward PH, House WF, Micevych PE, Bagger-Sjöbeck D. Re-evaluation of the role of the human indolymphatic sac in Ménière's disease. *Otolaryngol Head Neck Surg.* 1990;102:732–744.
34. Yuen SS, Schuknecht HF. Vestibular aqueduct and endolymphatic duct in Ménière's disease. *Arch Otolaryngol.* 1972;96:553–555.

5

Clinical Presentation of Ménière's Disease

John J. Chi, MD, and Michael J. Ruckenstein, MD

Introduction

Ménière's disease is characterized by intermittent episodes of vertigo lasting from minutes to hours with fluctuating sensorineural hearing loss, tinnitus, and aural pressure. Its diagnosis is primarily based on the clinical history, results of audiometric testing, and by ruling out other disorders that can present with similar symptoms. The disease is named for Prosper Ménière, who was among the first to propose that vertigo resulted from pathology within the inner ear, and not the central nervous system.[1] Ménière suggested that the episodic vertigo, ringing in the ears, and fluctuating hearing loss were associated with disease of the end organ of the inner ear. The classical history associated with a Ménière's attack was eloquently summarized by Barber.[2] Barber describes a patient of middle age and either sex, who initially develops unilateral aural fullness and tinnitus. These mild symptoms may persist or temporarily resolve, but ultimately, the patient develops an acute onset of severe unilateral aural fullness, roaring tinnitus, hearing loss, and rotary vertigo. The vertigo will last for a period of hours and may recur during the following days. Over time, the symptoms subside, leaving the patient with mild unsteadiness, tinnitus, and perhaps a mild hearing loss. Additional attacks will occur; however, the intervals between the attacks and their severity are unpredictable. In fact, the fluctuation, waxing, and waning of the symptoms of Ménière's disease is, in and of itself, a hallmark of the disorder.

Ménière's disease is a complex, progressive disease of the inner ear with a peculiar but characteristic presentation that can present diagnostic challenges to the clinician. The most recent definition of the disease has been established by the Committee on Hearing and Equilibrium of the American Academy of Otolaryngology-Head and Neck Surgery (AAO-HNS) (Table 5–1).[3] This chapter focuses on the clinical presentation of Ménière's disease, and provides the necessary foundation for the accurate diagnosis of this interesting, but enigmatic, disorder.

Epidemiology

The peculiar array of symptoms, and the oftentimes lack of coincident presentation, associated with Ménière's disease makes epidemiological analysis of the disease a difficult undertaking.[4] Patients may initially present with only vestibular symptoms, such as sudden onset vertigo, and be misdiagnosed with isolated vestibular dysfunction. Conversely, patients presenting with wholly auditory symptoms, such as hearing loss, tinnitus, or aural fullness, may be misdiagnosed with central nervous system disease or eustachian tube dysfunction. A paucity of publications exists in the scientific literature describing the epidemiology of Ménière's disease. Some studies suggest that males and females are equally affected by this disorder,[5–8] whereas others suggest a slight female prepon-

Table 5–1. AAO-HNS Criteria for the Diagnosis of Ménière's Disease (1995)[3]

Signs and Symptoms
• Recurrent spontaneous and episodic vertigo. A definitive spell of vertigo lasting at least 20 min, often prostrating, accompanied by dysequilibrium that can last several days; usually nausea or vomiting, or both; no loss of consciousness. Horizontal rotary nystagmus is always present • Hearing loss (not necessarily fluctuating) • Either aural fullness or tinnitus, or both
Classification
Certain Ménière's Disease • Definite disease with histopathologic confirmation **Definite Ménière's Disease** • Two or more definitive episodes of vertigo with hearing loss, plus tinnitus, aural fullness, or both **Probable Ménière's Disease** • Only one definitive episode of vertigo and the other symptoms and signs **Possible Ménière's Disease** • Definitive vertigo with no associated hearing loss or hearing loss with nondefinitive disequilibrium

derance of 1.3 to 1.[9] The onset of symptoms most frequently occurs during the fourth and fifth decade of life, with the first presentation rarely occurring before 20 years or after 70 years of age. Although rare, Ménière's disease has been described in the pediatric population.[10,11] Although population data on Ménière's disease is limited, Ménière's is predominantly a disease of caucasians of Northern European ancestry with an overall incidence of approximately 1 per 2,000.[12,13]

Auditory Symptoms

Sensorineural hearing loss is one of the defining signs of Ménière's disease. Ménière's disease typically presents with an up-sloping low-frequency hearing loss that over time often leads to a flat sensorineural hearing loss. In contrast to most other causes of sensorineural hearing loss (eg, noise, ototoxins, aging), the hearing loss associated with Ménière's disease typically begins as a low-frequency hearing loss. Additionally, profound sensorineural hearing loss associated with Ménière's disease is rare. Stahle found that 1 to 2% of patients with severe Ménière's disease developed profound hearing loss.[14] Total hearing loss should alert investigation of other possible causes for hearing loss (ie, central nervous system, syphilis, genetic, autoimmune).

The audiometric findings associated with Ménière's disease have been well described in the scientific literature with a special focus placed on the configuration of the audiogram. Several studies have noted one of two audiometric findings at the time of initial presentation. Patients usually present with either an isolated low-frequency sensorineural hearing loss or sensorineural hearing loss in the low (<2000 Hz) and high frequencies (>2000 Hz), with preservation of hearing in the middle frequency hearing (2000 Hz). The latter audiometric pattern is referred to as the inverted "V" audiogram or peaked pattern audiogram.[2,15] Stahle et al found that at the time of initial presentation, 28% of patients demonstrated an inverted "V" audiogram, 20% of patients had an isolated low-frequency hearing loss, and 21% of patients exhibited a flat hearing loss.[7] Katsarkis found that at initial presentation the magnitude of the hearing loss at lower frequencies was greater than that at higher frequencies.[8] Rarely, there also may be a slight conductive hearing loss noted at initial audiographical assessment,[16] which may lead to the misdiagnosis of eustachian tube dysfunction in patients presenting with early Ménière's disease.

Fluctuating hearing loss may be a prominent component of the clinical presentation, particularly in the early stages of the disease in patients with a low-frequency hearing loss. Although the literature describing fluctuation in hearing loss is limited, studies suggest that it may be present in 50 to 70% of patients with Ménière's disease.[5,6] Serial audiograms can document the characteristic fluctuation of sensorineural hearing loss.

The hearing loss associated with Ménière's disease progresses with advanced stages of the disease. Long-term follow-up studies suggest that hearing levels begin to stabilize approximately 5 years after the onset of symptoms. In the majority of patients, the audiogram eventually assumes a flat configuration and no longer fluctuates.[2,7] Stahle et al report a mean hearing loss of approximately 50 dB in the low and high frequencies.[7] In a series of over 100 patients followed for over 14 years, Green et al described a mean pure-tone average of 52 dB.[6] Katsarkis examined audiometric data from a large series of patients with Ménière's disease, many of whom were followed for over ten years, none of whom underwent surgical treatment, and found that slightly greater hearing loss remains in the lower frequencies.[8] Katsarkis found a mean threshold shift of approximately 40 dB at the lower frequencies and 30 dB at the higher frequencies. Although these studies followed large series of patients over a considerable period of time, the variation between patients must be taken into consideration when applying these findings in the clinical setting.

Other important auditory findings of Ménière's disease include hyperacusis and recruitment, diplacusis, tinnitus, and aural fullness. The hyperacusis experienced by patients with Ménière's disease is due to the recruitment of cochlear hair cells by the central nervous system and can be a particularly disturbing symptom.[2] As patients develop sensorineural hearing loss with progression of Ménière's disease, the onset of hypersensitivity to sounds can be stressful for both the patient and those around them. These symptoms may lead the patient to develop phonophobia. Diplacusis, the perception of the same tone at different pitches in the two ears, is another disconcerting symptom that has been described in Ménière's disease.[17] Recruitment and diplacusis arise from hair cell damage and are likely due to a loss of cochlear fine-tuning mechanisms. Paparella reported that recruitment and diplacusis occurred in 56% and 44% of Ménière's patients, respectively.[18] Tinnitus associated with Ménière's disease is another troubling symptom. The tinnitus is nonpulsatile with severity ranging from an intermittent loud roar, during an acute exacerbation, to a constant softer ringing sound, characteristic of Ménière's disease in its chronic stage.[19] Aural fullness is another symptom that presents with acute exacerbations of Ménière's disease. The incidence of this finding ranges from 50 to 70% and usually resolves with progression to chronic Ménière's disease.[5,6]

Vestibular Symptoms

The hallmark of Ménière's disease is episodic vertigo lasting from minutes to hours. This vertigo is described by patients as spinning vertigo in the horizontal axis that is often incapacitating. During episodes of acute exacerbation, the vertigo may occur on consecutive days, but no single episode lasts for more than 24 hours,[2] although the AAO-HNS criteria allows for disequilibrium that may persist for several days. Of note, de Sousa et al found that up to 50% of patients experiencing incapacitating vertigo may test normal on nystagmography and bithermal caloric assessments.[20] Typically, tinnitus and hearing loss precede and worsen with the onset of vertigo.

In addition to the vertigo, patients may experience nausea, vomiting, diaphoresis, and, most notably, horizontal nystagmus. The horizontal nystagmus during acute episodes of vertigo has been described in three phases: irritative, paralytic, and recovery. At the onset of the vertigo, the nystagmus is often in the direction of the affected ear—irritative nystagmus.[21] As the episode continues, the nystagmus beats away from the affected ear—paralytic nystagmus. At the end of the attack, as the vestibular system recovers function the nystagmus reverses again toward the affected ear—recovery nystagmus.[22,23]

During the early stages of Ménière's disease, episodes of vertigo can occur frequently—ranging from 6 to 11 attacks per year.[7] However, like the severity of hearing loss, the number of vertiginous episodes varies widely between patients. With disease progression to chronic Ménière's disease, the significance of the vertiginous episodes also declines. Shea described a system that characterizes the evolving symptomatology during Ménière's disease progression (Table 5–2).[24] Stahle et al reported that in patients with Ménière's disease for over 20 years, the incidence of vertiginous episodes decreased to three to four attacks per year. Green et al found a complete absence of vertigo or decrease in severity in 84% of patients followed over a period of nine years.[6] Of note, however: neither of these studies included data regarding the use of surgical interventions for treatment of the Ménière's disease in these patients. This proves to be an important omission in light of Silverstein's findings that approximately 50% of patients in whom surgical intervention was indicated experienced a resolution of symptoms without surgery.[25]

Psychological Symptoms of Ménière's Disease

Given the eccentric symptom complex of Ménière's disease and its profound effects on the patient's experience of the world, psychological manifestations of this disease would be expected to be more prevalent than the reported figures. A study of 120 patients presenting to an outpatient neurotology clinic found 42% of patients had psychopathology comorbid with their vestibular disease.[26] Coker et al investigated depression in patients with Ménière's disease and active vertigo using two different measures of depression and found a 70% to 80% incidence of depression.[27] However, in Ménière's patients without significant vertigo, the incidence

Table 5–2. Shea Staging System for Ménière's Disease

	I	*II*	*III*	*IV*	*V*
Fluctuant hearing loss	+	+			
Tinnitus	+	+	+	+	+
Aural fullness	+	+	+	+	
Vertigo		+	+		
Flat hearing loss			+	+	
Profound hearing loss					+

of depression was comparable to that of the control group. In a small series of patients with Ménière's disease and vestibular migraines, Eckhardt et al found psychopathology to be comorbid in 57% and 65% of patients, respectively.[28] Filipo et al also found that Ménière's patients had a higher incidence of dysphoria and somatization.[29] Additionally, Filipo reported that psychopathology was more prominent in patients requiring surgery and most prominent in patients that failed surgical therapy. Similarly, other longitudinal studies have shown that patients with organic vestibular disease comorbid with psychopathology are the ones most likely to remain symptomatic while also having the highest levels of handicap.[30,31] Whether the severity of Ménière's symptoms leads to more severe psychopathology, or vice versa, is not clear. Some authors suggest the latter and note that increased preexisting anxiety led to more severe Ménière's symptoms.[32–34] Hinchcliffe further suggested that Ménière's disease may be a psychosomatic disorder.[33] Conversely, Wexler and Crary suggested that the psychopathology is secondary to the Ménière's symptoms, and that the psychopathology has no role in the pathogenesis of this organic inner ear disease.[36]

Although an increased incidence of psychopathology in Ménière's disease is clear, the importance of this finding in understanding the pathogenesis of the disease remains controversial. However, the presence of depression, anxiety, and somatization in Ménière's patients warrants evaluation of the psychological symptoms in an effort to treat the Ménière's disease and improve the patient's overall quality of life.

Variants of Ménière's Disease

The clinical presentation of Ménière's disease can vary between patients, and the lack of coincident symptom presentation usually leads to auditory or vestibular symptoms predominating at the time of initial presentation. **Cochlear Ménière's disease** has been described as fluctuating hearing loss presenting in a patient in the absence of vestibular symptoms.[37] This presentation does not meet the AAO-HNS criteria for Ménière's disease and in the majority of patients represents the initial presentation of classical Ménière's disease. Because these patients are presenting with hearing loss, if vestibular symptoms do not ultimately develop, then it is imperative that another etiology of the hearing loss (ie, infectious, ototoxic, immune-mediated, genetic) be investigated. **Vestibular Ménière's disease** has been described as recurrent episodes of vertigo in the absence of auditory symptoms.[38] This presentation does not meet the AAO-HNS criteria for Ménière's disease and in a minority of patients, approximately 5 to 10%, represents the initial presentation of classical Ménière's disease.[39] The majority of these patients presenting with isolated vestibular symptoms do not have Ménière's disease but rather are most likely suffering from migrainous vertigo.[40]

The association between migraines, vertigo, and Ménière's disease has been an area of active research in recent years. Baloh suggested that Ménière's disease could potentially be the result of a "complication" of migraines in individuals genetically predisposed to migraines.[41] Baloh reported a series of six individuals with migraines and Ménière's disease, and suggested that the pathologic processes of migraines could damage the inner ear and predispose individuals for the development of Ménière's disease. Baloh also reported a study of eighteen patients with migraines and Ménière's disease that suggested an earlier onset of disease (37 years old) and a greater propensity for bilateral disease (56%).[42]

Bilateral Ménière's disease is a severe form of the disease with implications on quality of life and treatment. Long-term follow-up studies suggest that up to 50% of patients will eventually develop bilateral disease.[6–8,43]

Sudden falls without loss of consciousness, or drop attacks, have been associated with Ménière's disease. Tumarkin first described this entity in 1935.[44] The **otolithic crises of Tumarkin** are thought to be caused by acute utriculosaccular dysfunction, which leads to a sudden loss of extensor tone via the vestibulospinal pathway resulting in a fall. These attacks have been reported in 2 to 6% of Ménière's patients, occur in clusters, and self-resolve.[45,46] Ménière's patients presenting with drop attacks must be screened for other causes of drop attacks, such as vertebrobasilar insufficiency and migraines, using clinical history, physical examination, and appropriate radiologic studies.

In 1919, Lermoyez described a unique presentation of vertiginous spells in Ménière's patients. Typically, increasing tinnitus and hearing loss precede and worsen with the onset of vertigo. In **Lermoyez' syndrome** the preceding tinnitus and hearing loss resolve with the onset of vertigo.[47,48]

Conclusion

Ménière's disease is a chronic, progressive disorder that is defined and diagnosed based on the patient's clinical symptoms. It is hoped that the information provided in this chapter will be useful in facilitating an accurate clinical diagnosis.

References

1. Ménière P. Maladies de l'oreille interne offrant des symptoms de la congestion cerebral apoplectiforme. *Gaz Med de Paris.* 1961;16:88.
2. Barber HO. Ménière's disease: symptomatology. In: Oosterveld WJ, ed. *Ménière's Disease: A Comprehensive Appraisal.* New York, NY: John Wiley & Sons; 1983:25–34.
3. AAO-HNS 1995 Committee on Hearing and Equilibrium Guidelines for the Diagnosis and Evaluation of Therapy in Ménière's Disease. *Otolaryngol Head Neck Surg.* 1995;113:181–185.
4. da Costa S, de Sousa L, Piza M. Ménière's disease: overview, epidemiology, and natural history. *Otolaryngol Clin North Am.* 2002;35:455–495.
5. Haye R, Quist-Hanssen S. The natural course of Ménière's disease. *Acta Otolaryngol.* 1976;82:289–293.
6. Green J, Blum D, Harner S. Longitudinal followup of patients with Ménière's disease. *Otolaryngol Head Neck Surg.* 1991;104:783–788.
7. Stahle J, Friberg U, Svedberg A. Long-term progression of Ménière's disease. *Acta Otolaryngol Suppl.* 1991;485:78–83.
8. Katsarkis A. Hearing loss and vestibular dysfunction in Ménière's disease. *Acta Otolaryngol.* 1996;116:185–188.
9. da Costa S. Central causes of vertigo. In: Souza S, Claussen C, eds. *Modern*

Concepts of Neurology. Mumbai, India: Prajakta Arts,1997:310–331.
10. Paparella M, da Costa S, Fox R, Yoo T. Ménière's disease and other labyrinthine diseases. In: Paparella M, Shumrick D, Gluckmann J, Meyerhoff W, eds. *Otolaryngology.* 3rd ed. Philadelphia, PA: WB Saunders, 1991:1689–1714.
11. Meyerhoff W, Paparella M, Shea D. Ménière's disease in children. *Laryngoscope.* 1978;88:1504–1511.
12. Morrison A, Johnson K. Genetics and Ménière's disease. *Otolaryngol Clin North Am.* 2002;35:497–516.
13. Friberg U, Stahle J. The epidemiology of Ménière's disease. In: Harris J, ed. *Ménière's Disease.* The Hague, Netherlands: Kugler Publications; 1999:17–28.
14. Stahle J. Advanced Ménière's disease: a study of 356 severely disabled patients. *Acta Otolaryngol.* 1976;81:113–119.
15. Paparella M, McDermott J, de Sousa L. Ménière's disease and the peak audiogram. *Arch Otolaryngol.* 1982;108:555–559.
16. Arts H, Kileny P, Telian S. Diagnostic testing for endolymphatic hydrops. *Otolaryngol Clin North Am.* 1997;30: 987–1005.
17. Brookes G, Coelho A. Binaural diplacusis in Ménière's disease. In: Filipo R, Barbara M, eds. *Ménière's Disease: Perspectives in the '90s.* Amsterdam/New York: Kugler Publishing, 1994:31–37.
18. Paparella, M. The cause and pathogenesis of Ménière's disease and its symptoms. *Acta Otolaryngol.* 1985;99:445–451.
19. Vernon J, Johnson R, Schleuning A. The characteristics and natural history of tinnitus in Ménière's disease. *Otolaryngol Clin North Am.* 1980;13:611–619.
20. de Sousa L, Piza M, da Costa S. Diagnosis of Ménière's disease: routine and extended tests. *Otolaryngol Clin North Am.* 2002;35:547–564.
21. Bance M. The changing direction of nystagmus in acute Ménière's disease: pathophysiological implications. *Laryngoscope.* 1991;101:197–201.
22. Brown D, McClure J, Downar-Zapolski Z. The membrane rupture theory of Ménière's disease: is it valid? *Laryngoscope.* 1988;98:599–601.
23. McClure J, Copp J, Lyett P. Recovery nystagmus in Ménière's disease. *Laryngoscope.* 1981;91:1727–1737.
24. Shea J, Ge X. Streptomycin perfusion of the labyrinth through the round window plus intravenous streptomycin. *Otolaryngol Clin N Am.* 1994;27:317–324.
25. Silverstein H, Smouha E, Jones R. Natural history vs. surgery for Ménière's disease. *Otolaryngol Head Neck Surg.* 1989;100:6–15.
26. McKenna L, Hallam R, Hinchcliffe R. The prevalence of psychological disturbance in neurootology outpatients. *Clin Otolaryngol.* 1991;16:452–456.
27. Coker N, Coker R, Jenkins H, et al. Psychological profile of patients with Ménière's disease. *Arch Otolaryngol Head Neck Surg.* 1989;115:1355–1357.
28. Eckhardt-Henn A, Best C, Bense S, et al. Psychiatric comorbidity in different organic vertigo syndromes. *J Neurol.* 2008;255:420–428.
29. Filipo R, Lazzari R, Barbara M, et al. Psychological evolution of patients with Ménière's disease in relation to therapy. *Am J Otol.* 1988;9:306–309.
30. Godemann F, Koffroth C, Neu P, Heuser I. Why does vertigo become chronic after neuropathia vestibularis? *Psychosom Med.* 2004;66:783–787.
31. Silberstein S, Lipton R, Breslau N. Migraine: association with personality characteristics and psychopathology. *Cephalalgia.* 1995;15:358–369.
32. Fowler E, Zeckel A. Psychophysiological factors in Ménière's disease. *Psychosom Med.* 1953;15:127–139.
33. Hinchcliffe R. Personality profile in Ménière's disease. *J Laryngol Otol.* 1967; 81:477–481.
34. Lucente F. Psychiatric problems in otolaryngology. *Ann Otol Rhinol Laryngol.* 1973;82:340–346.

35. Hinchcliffe R. Emotion as a precipitating factor in Ménière's disease. *J Laryngol Otol.* 1967;81:471–475.
36. Wexler M, Crary W. Ménière's disease: the psychosomatic hypothesis. *Am J Otol.* 1986;7:93–96.
37. Shea J. Definition of fluctuant hearing loss. *Otolaryngol Clin North Am.* 1975;8: 263–266.
38. Paparella M, Mancini F. Vestibular Ménière's disease. *Otolaryngol Head Neck Surg.* 1985;93:148–151.
39. LeLiever W, Barber H. Recurrent vestibulopathy. *Laryngoscope.* 1981;91:1–6.
40. Rassekh C, Harker L. The prevalence of migraine in Ménière's disease. *Laryngoscope.* 1992;102:135–138.
41. Cha Y, Kane M, Baloh R. Familial clustering of migraine, episodic vertigo, and Ménière's disease. *Otol Neurotol.* 2008;29:93–96.
42. Cha Y, Brodsky J, Ishiyama G, Sabatti C, Baloh R. The relevance of migraine in patients with Ménière's disease. *Acta Otolaryngol.* 2007;127:1241–1245.
43. Paparella M, Sajjadi H. Natural history of Ménière's disease. In: Harris J, ed. *Ménière's Disease.* The Hague, Netherlands: Kugler Publications. 1999:29–38.
44. Tumarkin A. The otolithic catastrophe. *Br Med J.* 1936;2:135–138.
45. Baloh R, Jacobson K, Winder T. Drop attacks with Ménière's syndrome. *Ann Neurol.* 1990;28:384–387.
46. Janzen D, Russell RD. Conservative management of Tumarkin's otolithic crisis. *J Otolaryngol.* 1988;17:359–361.
47. Lermoyez M. Le vertige qui fait entendre (angiospasme labyrinthique). *Presse Med.* 1919;27:1.
48. Pillsbury H, Postma D. Lermoyez' syndrome and the otolithic crisis of Tumarkin. *Otolaryngol Clin North Am.* 1983;16: 197–203.

6

Differential Diagnosis

Jason Liebowitz, MD and
Michael J. Ruckenstein, MD

Introduction

There are numerous disorders that can present in a fashion similar to Ménière's. This section provides a brief overview of the disease processes included in the differential diagnosis of Ménière's disease, in order to provide the clinician with a framework to diagnose and manage these processes.

Congenital Problems

Definition

Congenital malformations of the membranous or osseomembranous components of the inner ear result from defects in inner ear development during the fourth through eighth week of fetal gestation.

Incidence

The overall incidence of congenital inner ear deformities cannot be determined directly because only bony abnormalities of the inner ear can be detected by imaging. The overall incidence of congenital hearing loss is 1 to 3 per 1,000 live births.[1] Risk factors associated with congenital hearing loss include: greater than two-day NICU admission, syndromic hearing loss, family history of hereditary hearing loss, craniofacial abnormalities, and congenital infections.[2] The majority of these patients have no radiographic abnormalities of the inner ear, and are felt to have abnormalities affecting the membranous labyrinth.

Etiology

Studies from animal models of hereditary hearing loss indicate that congenital inner ear disorders result from a defect in the genetic mechanism that controls labyrinthine organogenesis.[3] In most human cases of bony labyrinthine anomalies, this appears to be sporadic. Rarely, these mutations may cause abnormalities in more than one organ system, resulting in a syndromic presentation.[4] In most cases, the factors causing the genetic mutation remain obscure; however, chemical (eg, thalidomide) and infectious (rubella, cytomegalovirus) teratogens have been noted to cause bony labyrinthine abnormalities, and familial patterns of inheritance have rarely been identified.[5–7] Membranous abnormalities (cochleosaccular Scheibe degeneration) are most commonly associated with hereditary patterns of hearing loss.

Pathology

Jackler and colleagues developed a logical categorization of congenital inner ear anomalies based on the known sequence of labyrinthine organogenesis.[8] This classification system divides abnormalities into membranous and osseomembranous categories.

Clinical Presentation

Hearing loss is the primary presenting symptom. Hearing loss may be present at birth or may develop within the first two decades of life. The hearing loss may vary from mild to profound, and may be progressive or fluctuating. The incidence of vestibular dysfunction in this patient population has not been well documented and is largely unknown. In one study, 20% of patients with congenital ear anomalies complained of vertigo or imbalance. In general, children with decreased or absent vestibular function rarely show evidence of fluctuating vestibular function, but present with general "clumsiness" and delay in gross motor skills (such as walking).[9]

Investigations

Congenital anomalies of the otic capsule typically are diagnosed with high resolution CT scan of the temporal bone, which allows for careful assessment of the inner ear structures. MRI is used in addition to CT scanning, especially prior to cochlear implantation, to document the presence of fluid within the membranous labyrinth, to identify the cochlear division of the eighth cranial nerve, and to evaluate adjacent brain structures.[10] Abnormalities on vestibular testing are frequently recorded in patients with congenital inner ear deformities; however, these patients often do not manifest complaints related to vestibular function. There is no clear consensus in the literature regarding routine vestibular testing of patients with congenital hearing loss.[9,11,12]

Treatment

Hearing amplification, with conventional hearing aids or cochlear implants is the mainstay of treatment. Vestibular rehabilitation assists in recovery from an uncompensated vestibular loss. Children with bilateral vestibular loss are taught substitutive sensory and motor strategies, although most children eventually acquire balance control without any vestibular rehabilitation.[9] Patients are counseled to avoid dangerous situations in which the proprioceptive and visual systems are impaired (ie, swimming in the dark). Patients with identified osseomembranous anomalies are cautioned against activities that may predispose to head trauma.

Prognosis

Studies now document the efficacy of cochlear implantation in this patient population. Vestibular complaints are self-limited, with patients adapting well to their peripheral vestibular loss. This may be due to the excellent plasticity of the immature brain, as well as compensation by the visual and somatosensory systems.[13]

Trauma—Temporal Bone

Definition

Both blunt and penetrating trauma to the temporal bone can cause damage to the inner ear or VIIIth cranial nerve, resulting in sensorineural hearing loss and vertigo.

Incidence and Etiology

Head injuries occur in approximately 75% of motor vehicle accidents, with approximately 20% of these patients displaying some symptoms related to temporal bone trauma.[14,15] The majority of injuries are unilateral, with bilateral fractures reported in 9 to 20% of cases.[16] Motor vehicle accidents are the most common cause of blunt trauma to the temporal bone (45%), followed by falls (20%), altercations (10%), and athletic injuries (10%). Penetrating trauma is a less common form of temporal bone injury. Etiologies range from gunshot wounds to cotton swab injuries.

Pathology

Temporal bone fractures have classically been defined by their relationship to the long axis of the temporal bone. Longitudinal fractures pass along the external auditory canal, through the tegmen of the middle ear, and then pass anterior to the bony labyrinth to terminate at either the foramen lacerum or spinosum.

Transverse fractures run perpendicular to the long axis of the temporal bone. They transverse the petrous apex between the foramen magnum and the foramen lacerum or spinosum, typically disrupting the bony labyrinth or the internal auditory canal. However, the majority of temporal bone fractures fail to follow these traditional classifications, but are a mixture of both. They are classified as oblique or mixed temporal bone fractures.

More recently, temporal bone fractures have been classified radiographically as otic-capsule violating or otic capsule sparing; this classification appears to be the most predictive of outcome and correlates well with facial nerve injury, sensorineural hearing loss, and CSF otorrhea.[17,18] Depending on their trajectory, penetrating projectiles may involve any or all aspects of the temporal bone.

Clinical Presentation

The hallmark of labyrinthine injury secondary to blunt or penetrating trauma is the presence of vertigo and hearing loss. Because of the immense force required to produce a temporal bone fracture, patients usually have multiple injuries and present with associated nontemporal skull fractures (47%), maxillofacial fractures (21%), orthopedic injuries outside of the head and neck (16%), cervical spine injury (2–6%), and intracranial injury (up to 84%).[16] Other associated injuries include facial nerve paralysis, CSF leak, vascular injury, and cranial nerve palsies. In cases of severe head trauma, the patient may report imbalance (as opposed to vertigo) if they have been comatose for a period of time. Even in fractures that do not cause direct injury to the inner ear or eighth cranial nerve, patients may still suffer sensorineural hearing loss or vertigo due to labyrinthine concussion. Labyrinthine concussion typically results in acute self-limited vertigo, and the hearing loss is, at least, partially reversible. In contrast, fractures that affect the otic capsule or internal auditory canal result in profound hearing loss and vertigo. Signs on physical exam include a tuning fork test that lateralizes to the unaffected ear and spontaneous nystagmus consistent with either an irritative (toward affected ear) or paretic (away from the affected ear) lesion.

Investigations

Audiometric and vestibular testing confirms the presence of inner ear pathology and delineate the degree of damage. High-resolution CT scan (noncontrast, 0.5 to 0.75-mm cuts[19]) of the temporal bone is indicated to define the nature of the fracture and the structures involved. MRI is the imaging modality of choice to evaluation of acute facial nerve palsy and sensorineural hearing loss.

Treatment

Other than for perilymphatic fistula, no specific treatment exists for penetrating or blunt temporal bone trauma. Vestibular suppressants can be used for acute vertigo control if not contraindicated by the patient's overall medical status. Hearing aid amplification may be beneficial in patients with partial sensorineural hearing loss. Cochlear implantation is an option for patients with profound sensorineural hearing loss following temporal bone trauma; however, the rate of facial nerve stimulation is increased.[20] There is benefit from the BAHA in acquired unilateral sensorineural hearing loss.[21] Vestibular rehabilitation is indicated in patients with a slow recovery from their vestibular loss. Some patients may develop delayed posttraumatic vertigo and hearing loss analogous to Ménière's disease. Treatment is similar to that of Ménière's disease. Benign positional vertigo (BPPV) commonly develops days to weeks after trauma due to displacement of otoconia; treatment with repositioning maneuvers is usually curative.[16]

Prognosis

Most patients sustaining temporal bone injuries develop little or no inner ear dysfunction. Patients who do sustain an uncompensated vestibular loss generally respond well to vestibular rehabilitation. Sequela of temporal bone injury include BPPV, meningocele, encephalocele, cholesteatoma, CSF leak, and meningitis.

Barotrauma

Definition

Subjecting the inner ear to rapid and significant changes in ambient pressure may result in temporary or permanent inner ear dysfunction.

Incidence and Etiology

All forms of inner ear barotrauma are rare. The most common etiology is diving (some report up to a 33% incidence of inner ear decompression trauma in divers with decompression sickness[22] and 14% of divers in general[23]), although airplane flights and forceful sneezing may cause pathology as well.

Pathology and Pathogenesis

Alternobaric trauma (middle ear barotrauma) is the most benign of these entities.[24] It occurs during ascent during a dive or an airplane flight, resulting in temporary vertigo or sensorineural hearing loss. Asymmetric middle ear pressure between the two ears is thought to be required to elicit symptoms. The underlying pathogenic mechanism is unknown.

Atmospheric inner ear trauma typically occurs in divers or may occur after a forceful sneeze.[25–27] This is thought to occur due to rapid pressure changes of the inner ear, and may often be permanent. Such pressure changes may result in labyrinthine concussion (temporary dysfunction with no anatomic correlate due to metabolic abnormalities), intralabyrinthine membrane tears, intralabyrinthine bleeding, or damage to receptor cells. In its most extreme form it may result in a perilymphatic fistula. Inner ear barotraumas is usually associated with alternobaric trauma of the middle ear due to underlying eustachian tube dysfunction.[23]

Inner ear decompression sickness is believed to result from gas bubbles precipitating in the labyrinthine fluids and vessels.[28] It occurs due to rapid pressure changes (rapid reduction in ambient pressure). It usually occurs in cases when patients have dived to a depth of >15 meters for >20 minutes.[23] It can lead to permanent damage to the inner ear, which may be secondary to ischemia. There is an increased risk in divers with a right to left vascular shunt; this is thought to be due to venous gas emboli crossing over into the arterial system.[22]

Clinical Presentation

Vertigo is the most common presenting symptom, and may be associated with decreased hearing. Alternobaric trauma is associated with rapid resolution upon equilibration of the middle ear pressure. By the time the patient seeks medical attention, the examination and investigation is usually normal.

Atmospheric inner ear trauma may present with vertigo, hearing loss, tinnitus, or nausea and vomiting. These symptoms persist after the exposure, as opposed to middle ear barotraumas.

The vertigo is usually described as more of a feeling of instability or slight dizziness. Klingmann et al report a higher incidence of hearing loss in this patient population with only 35% of patients reporting vertigo or disequilibrium (usually described as instability or slight dizziness).[23] Tuning fork tests and audiometric assessment reveals a sensorineural hearing loss of variable severity. Nystagmus, of the irritative or paretic variety, also may be observed.

Nearly all cases of inner ear decompression sickness present with vertigo as the initial symptom; it may be accompanied by hearing loss or tinnitus, which tends to appear at a later time when the vertiginous symptoms have subsided.[23] The presentation may be identical to that of atmospheric inner ear trauma; it is clinically differentiated from atmospheric inner ear pressure due to its temporal relationship with a rapid ascent from a dive as well as other associated symptoms of acute decompression sickness such as "the bends."

Investigations

Audiometric evaluation is required in all forms of barotrauma. Vestibular function may be indicated in patients with persistent symptoms.

Treatment

Alternobaric trauma requires no specific treatment other than encouraging equilibration of middle ear pressure during flight.

Patients with atmospheric inner ear barotraumas are initially managed with bed rest, head elevation and avoidance of straining.[25] Some advocate high dose steroids as well as nasal decongestion and rheologic therapy (ie, pentoxyfillin).[23] Patients with persistent symptoms of fluctuating hearing loss or vertigo may require middle ear exploration for perilymphatic fistula. Patients are also counseled to avoid straining and further pressure changes that may exacerbate symptoms.

Patients with inner ear decompression trauma require immediate recompression in a hyperbaric oxygen chamber. Some also advocate steroids as well as rheologic therapy.[23]

Prognosis

Alternobaric trauma carries an excellent prognosis. Atmospheric and inner ear decompression trauma may result in variable degrees of permanent hearing and vestibular loss.

Perilymphatic Fistula

Definition

A perilymphatic fistula (PLF) occurs when the boundary between the middle ear and inner ear has been violated, allowing egress of perilymph and resulting in inner ear dysfunction.

Incidence, Etiology, and Pathology

Perilymphatic fistulas are proposed to occur via three possible mechanisms. Congenital inner ear anomalies involving the otic capsule may result in dehiscences in the labyrinth that allow for communication between the middle ear and labyrinth. The typical presentation is that of severe to profound hearing loss and recurrent meningitis or CSF leak.[29]

PLF also may result from disruption of the oval or round window due to external trauma. The trauma may be iatrogenic (eg, poststapes surgery) or secondary to blunt or penetrating trauma.[30] There are two major mechanisms of PLF following trauma: explosive and implosive. Explosive trauma results from increased pressure in the CSF being transmitted to the perilymphatic space; implosive trauma is due to pressure applied to the oval window or round window.[31] In addition, barotraumas and acoustic trauma have both been proposed as possible etiologic factors due to transmission of rapid pressure changes to the round and oval window.[32] As indicated previously, these forms of trauma rarely result in a frank PLF.

Most of the controversy surrounding PLF pertains to the spontaneous variety. This is proposed to arise from a congenital dehiscence in the region of the oval or round window; this may be precipitated by an increase in intracranial pressure being transmitted to the inner ear (explosive trauma). The validity of the concept of spontaneous PLF has been critically scrutinized by otologists over the past few years with a consensus emerging among most authorities that spontaneous fistulas rarely, if ever, occur.[33,34]

Clinical Presentation

PLF may present with various symptoms common to other otologic diseases, specifically Ménière's disease, including hearing loss, vertigo, and tinnitus. The diagnosis is more readily apparent when these symptoms occur in a temporal relationship to a precipitating traumatic event. Fluctuations in hearing may support the diagnosis if they appear provoked by pressure fluctuations or straining.

Investigations

No valid or accurate diagnostic test exists for PLF. The fistula test may be positive in cases of PLF; however, this test is nonspecific and may be positive in other conditions such as Ménière's disease and otosyphilis. Its utility in diagnosis is debated in the literature.[35,36] Audiovestibular testing, including electronystagmography and electrocochleography, does not reveal any pathognomonic findings. Despite its utility in CSF leaks, detection of fluorescein in the middle ear after IV or intrathecal administration has not proven to be clinically useful. This may be due to the small amount of fluid leakage into the middle ear.

Similarly, the detection of beta-2 transferrin in the middle ear has not proven to be an accurate method for detection of PLF.[37] This is likely a direct result of the dilutional effect during sample preparation, dilution in middle ear fluid, or dilution in preoperative injection fluids prior to sample collection (all of which lower the concentration of beta-2 transferrin below detectable levels).[38] The utility of radiographic imaging is in excluding other conditions; current imaging techniques are not reliable for detection of PLF.

Most authorities agree that the only reliable method of detection is direct observation of leakage.[35] There is evidence to suggest that the most accurate way of exploration is endoscopic via the tympanic membrane (endoscopic visualization of fluid leakage via a myringotomy).[39,40] This technique appears to avoid false positive results that occur secondary to pooling of fluid, such as anesthetic injection, during traditional exploration methods utilizing a tympanomeatal flap.

Treatment

Bed rest, head elevation, and avoidance of straining are the initial treatments for suspected PLF. Symptomatic treatment can be used for patients with severe bouts of vertigo. If symptoms of fluctuating hearing loss or vertigo persist beyond 2 or 3 days despite conservative management, middle ear exploration with patching of the fistula site should be considered. Some advocate for patching of both the oval and round window regardless of whether a leak is seen at a single window.[31]

Prognosis

Some fistulas heal spontaneously. There is no clear literature detailing the incidence of need for exploration. Friedland and Wackym summarized the surgical outcomes from multiple institutions. Overall, of patients requiring surgical exploration, approximately 90% have an improvement in vestibular symptoms, approximately 50% stabilization of hearing, and improvement in hearing in approximately 15% following exploration.[34] In patients who sustain a frank stapes subluxation from external trauma, the prognosis is more guarded for return of auditory function.

Metabolic—Otosclerosis

Definition

Otosclerosis is a genetic and metabolic disease of the bone of the otic capsule.

Incidence and Etiology

Otosclerosis is present at autopsy in approximately 10% of Caucasians; however, it is clinically manifest in only 1% of this population.[41,42] The incidence in African Americans is approximately one-tenth that of the Caucasian population; it is virtually nonexistent in Native Americans. Although the incidence of pathology at autopsy is equivalent in males and females, clinical symptoms are twice as likely to occur in females.

Otosclerosis appears to follow an autosomal dominant pattern of inheritance with a penetrance rate of 25% to 40%, although the precise mode of inheritance has not been definitively elucidated.[43,44] A plethora of research aimed at defining the underlying genetic mutation has not identified a causative gene, although eight potential otosclerosis loci have been identified to date.[43,45,46] Some authors have attempted to link otosclerosis with the HLA region of chromosome 6 coding for the major histocompatibility complex; to date, there is no definitive proof of an association.[43]

Earlier studies have identified measles virus gene products within the otosclerotic foci as well as mutations in the collagen type I gene (COL1A1 gene), a genetic defect also identified in mild forms of osteogenesis imperfecta, as causative factors for the development of otosclerosis.[47,48] These authors speculate that the development of otosclerosis may involve the localization of a measles infection within the otic capsule. In patients with the appropriate genetic defect, this infection may precipitate the abnormal bone turnover characteristic of otosclerosis.

More recent research has shown that mutation in COL1A1 has only a mild effect on susceptibility to otosclerosis.[49]

Pathology

Otosclerosis progresses from an initial spongiotic phase characterized by hypervascularity and osteoclastic bone resorption through a sclerotic phase, characterized by deposition of dense lamellar bone.[50] These processes appear to occur preferentially at certain sites, such as the fissula ante fenestram (at the anterior lip of the oval window), as well as in close proximity to the round window. Involvement of the fissula ante fenestram results in characteristic stapes fixation and conductive hearing loss.

Foci of otosclerosis along the lateral cochlear wall appear to cause degeneration of the adjacent spiral ligament and stria vascularis.[51] Degeneration of outer hair cells has also been observed. This appears to account for the sensorineural hearing loss seen in a subset of patients with otosclerosis. Vestibular symptoms appear to be the result of degeneration of vestibular nerve afferent fibers, which are not in the direct proximity of the otosclerotic foci.[52]

Clinical Presentation

Otosclerosis typically presents in young to middle age individuals who complain of slowly progressive hearing loss (typically bilateral) and tinnitus. The hearing loss is typically conductive.

Studies report a variable incidence of vestibular complaints in these patients. In addition, the manner in which the symptoms are described is not standardized, making it difficult to discern the precise nature of vestibular complaints. With this in mind, it is possible to state the following with regards to otosclerosis and vestibular complaints. Most patients with vestibular complaints complain of vertigo, while a minority complain of imbalance. Vertiginous patients manifest three possible patterns of presentation. Positional vertigo is a complaint in a significant number of patients.[52] A small number present with complaints akin to Ménière's disease (fluctuating, mixed or SNHL with episodic vertigo).[53] A third group, referred to as McCabe as otosclerotic inner ear syndrome, presents with recurrent episodes of vertigo with nonfluctuating conductive hearing loss.[54,55] Some of these cases may actually be attributable to superior semicircular canal dehiscence syndrome.[56,57]

Although typically presenting with a conductive hearing loss, sensorineural hearing loss is a common finding in these patients, particularly later in the disorder.[51,58] In a minority of patients, sensorineural hearing loss may be the dominant form of hearing loss. Complaints of vestibular dysfunction have been documented in 10 to 46% of patients.[52–55,59] The presence of vestibular complaints appears to correlate with the degree of sensorineural hearing loss.

Investigations

Otosclerosis has been referred to as the condition in which the patient hears nothing and the physician sees nothing. Other than abnormalities in the tuning fork tests, the examination typically is normal. A subset of patients may display a Schwartze sign, a red hue on the promontory and oval window niche, characteristic of increased vascularity due to active bone resorption. Audiometric evaluation typically reveals a bilateral conductive or mixed hearing loss pattern. Hallmark findings include Carhart's notch (decreased bone conduction threshold at 2000 Hz) and paracusis of Willis (improvement of hearing with increased background noise).

A variety of abnormalities consistent with peripheral disease may be noted on vestibular testing, most notably a reduction in caloric response. CT scan may reveal evidence of lucency within the otic capsule, indicative of cochlear otosclerosis. Its use in diagnosis of otosclerosis is limited.

Treatment

Stapedectomy remains the treatment of choice for otosclerosis. Hearing aid amplification is a therapeutic alternative, particularly in cases of mixed or sensorineural hearing loss. Cochlear implantation also is an alternative in profound hearing loss, although there is an increased rate of facial nerve stimulation.[60]

Most patients with vestibular complaints note that these symptoms resolved after stapedectomy.[55] The use of fluoride for otosclerosis has been heavily debated in the literature. Some advocate for its use in nonsurgical candidates or those with sensorineural hearing loss or vestibular complaints. However, its efficacy has never been established in patients with vestibular complaints.[61]

Prognosis

Significant vestibular complaints occur only in a minority of patients with otosclerosis. Most of these patients appear to be well controlled with medical or surgical interventions. For those with positional vertigo, vestibular and balance rehabilitation programs may offer symptomatic relief.

Neoplasm

Definition

Neoplastic lesions causing auditory and vestibular pathology may occupy the cerebellopontine angle (CPA) or the petrous apex.

Incidence and Epidemiology

Vestibular schwannoma (acoustic neuroma) are the most common lesion in this category, with a reported incidence of approximately 10 to 13 adults per million per year.[62–64] The true incidence, however, may actually be higher, with a reported incidence of unsuspected vestibular schwannoma in 0.7% of brain MRI studies.[65] The majority occur sporadically (95%); approximately 5% occur as part of neurofibromatosis type 2 syndrome and are characteristically bilateral.

Meningiomas are the most common benign brain tumor, accounting for 13 to 20% of all intracranial neoplasms, of which 3 to 8% occupy the petroclival region or CPA.[66] Other rare tumors affecting the CPA include epidermoids, lipomas, primary brain neoplasms (gliomas, astrocytoma, ependymomas, and carcinomatous meningitis), schwannomas from other cranial nerves, and metastatic lesions.

Lesions of the petrous apex are rare. Those most common resulting in cochleovestibular pathology include cholesterol granulomas (truly an inflammatory lesion) and epidermoids.[67] Other lesions that can affect the petrous apex and rarely lead to cochleovestibular pathology include cranial nerve schwannomas, clival cordomas, glomus jugulare tumors, and sarcomas.

Pathology

Vestibular schwannomas may arise either at the Obersteiner-Redlich zone of the vestibular nerve (the junction of central and peripheral myelin) or from the schwann cell population of the vestibular ganglion.[68] Histopathologic analysis reveals the classic Antoni A and Antoni B patterns. These tumors grow medially, filling the internal auditory canal (IAC), the CPA, and ultimately compressing the contents of the posterior fossa. Mutations in a tumor suppressor gene on chromosome 22 (NF2 gene) are associated with tumors arising in patients with NF2 and in sporadic vestibular schwannomas.[7,69,70] The rate of mutation of the NF2 gene is higher in sporadic cases than in NF2 cases.[71]

Meningiomas arise from cap cells that cluster at the tips of arachnoid villi.[72] They grow along the dura overlying the posterior face of the petrous bone, involving the contents of the IAC and the clivus, as well as the contents of the posterior cranial fossa.

Cholesterol granulomas of the petrous apex are inflammatory cystic lesions that form in well-pneumatized temporal bones.[73] They were thought to arise when aeration of the air cell tracts become obstructed, forming a vacuum and ultimately causing hemorrhage from mucosal vessels. A more recent hypothesis has proposed that the lesions do not form from a hemorrhage due to vacuum formation in air cell tracts, but rather due to clival bone marrow rests that become sequestered in well pneumatized temporal bones.[73] Breakdown products of the hemorrhagic exudates or from marrow secretions, including cholesterol, incite an inflammatory response that results in an expansile cystic lesion that can erode surrounding osseous structures, including the labyrinth. Primary epidermoid tumors arise from squamous rests and possess the same characteristics on histopathologic analysis as cholesteotomas.[74]

Clinical Presentation

Although vestibular schwannomas originate on the vestibular portion of the VIIIth cranial nerve, most (>90%) patients present with hearing loss and tinnitus. Imbalance, particularly in the dark, occurs in 50% of patients, whereas 20% of patients have vertigo. Paresthesias or pain in the trigeminal distribution occur in up to 50% of patients, whereas facial nerve dysfunction (typically twitching) occurs in approximately 10%. Very large tumors may cause cerebellar ataxia;

however, early recognition of tumors afforded by MRI imaging has reduced the incidence of these large lesions.[75–77]

Meningiomas of the CPA present with similar symptoms to vestibular schwannomas; however, they differ in the frequency of these symptoms being present.[78,79] Only 60% of patients present with hearing loss, but facial pain is considerably more common (60%). These tumors also have a higher incidence of cerebellar compression.

Cholesterol granulomas most commonly present with pain, headache, and diplopia.[80,81] Otalgia, vertigo, hearing loss, and Vth nerve paresthesias are other common presenting complaints. In contrast, epidermoids of the petrous apex most commonly present with hearing loss and facial paralysis.[74] Vertigo is a less common complaint in patients with these lesions.

Investigations

Audiometric assessment reveals sensorineural hearing loss of variable degrees in cases of intracranial lesions (vestibular schwannomas, meningiomas). Meningiomas tend to be larger than vestibular schwannomas before precipitating hearing loss. Lesions of the petrous apex may cause a sensorineural or mixed hearing loss depending on what structures are involved. Vestibular testing can reveal a wide variety of results depending on the size of the tumor. Intracranial tumors that encroach on the VIIIth cranial nerve demonstrate signs of peripheral vestibular lesions, most commonly a reduction in caloric response. At the bedside, one may observe hyperventilation induced nystagmus, typically beating to the side of the lesion. As tumors encroach on the brainstem and cerebellum, central signs on oculomotor testing, as well as central patterns of nystagmus, may be evident.

Lesions of the CPA and posterior fossa are most accurately diagnosed with MR imaging with gadolinium enhancement. Limited MR imaging scans, typically T2-weighted fast spin echo scans, may prove to be a cost-effective and accurate method of screening for retrocochlear pathology.[82,83] Auditory brainstem response (ABR) audiometry has a limited role in screening for retrocochlear pathology; its role is largely historical.[84] In patients who cannot undergo MRI, CT with contrast is a reasonable alternative.

Petrous apex lesions are typically evaluated with both CT and MRI.[67] CT scans of cholesterol granulomas and epidermoids reveal nonenhancing expansile lesions; cholesterol granulomas are highly pneumatized while epidermoids are not. These lesions can be differentiated on MRI by the fact that epidermoids are hypointense on T1 and cholesterol granulomas are hyperintense on T1 (both lesions are bright on T2 and neither lesion enhances with gadolinium).

Treatment

Traditionally, surgical excision via a hearing preservation (retrosigmoid, middle fossa) or hearing ablative (translabyrinthine) approach was the treatment of choice for tumors of the CPA. Surgery continues to be a mainstay of treatment; however, stereotactic radiosurgery alone or in the adjuvant setting (ie, gamma knife) or fractionated stereotactic radiation therapy are alternative treatment options, with the theoretical advantage of achieving tumor control with smaller tumors while minimizing morbidity and cost.[85]

Most authors favor drainage procedures for cholesterol granulomas using hearing preservation approaches (infralabyrinthine, infracochlear).[81,86] In some cases, it is necessary to excise these lesions. Epidermoids are challenging lesions to excise, as they tend to adhere to a variety of intracranial structures that make total excision difficult.[74] Clival cordomas that invade the petrous apex represent a similar surgical challenge. Postsurgical vestibular and balance rehabilitation programs can be very effective in the management of residual symptoms.

Prognosis

Other than the rare malignant lesion, the prognosis of patients with these lesions is fairly good. The advent of MRI, allowing for the detection of smaller tumors, and the development of improved skull base approaches and treatment options, has decreased major complication rates and improved hearing preservation. The popularization of drainage procedures for cholesterol granulomas has allowed most of these lesions to be treated adequately with minimal morbidity.

Infectious—Syphilis

Definition

Systemic infection by *Treponema pallidum* may be transmitted transplacentally or may be contracted via sexual contact. Syphilis is a systemic disease characterized by classic stages interspersed with periods lacking significant symptoms. Sensorineural hearing loss has been reported in secondary and late syphilis.

Incidence and Epidemiology

The incidence of syphilis peaked in the United States in the 1940s. In 2000, the rate of primary and secondary syphilis was 2.1 per 100,000. Recently, there has been an increasing incidence of syphilitic infection, specifically in the male homosexual population and the HIV-positive population.[87] It may be present in up to 7% on patients thought to have Ménière's disease.[88] Hearing loss is present in 40% of patients with congenital syphilis and up to 80 to 90% of patients with neurosyphilis.[89]

Pathology

The changes in the inner ear resulting from syphilis have been well described. The otic capsule may be involved during the secondary and/or tertiary stages of infection. Involvement manifests as osteitis of the otic capsule bone.[50] Inflammation is mediated by mononuclear cells, and results in patchy bone resorption; these spaces are subsequently filled with fatty marrow and loose connective tissue.[90] It is accompanying by an obliterate endarteritis typical of syphilitic infection. In severe cases, gumma (lymphocytic infiltrates, vascular occlusion, and central necrosis) may be noted in the otic capsule. In addition, degeneration of the labyrinthine membrane, endolymphatic hydrops, and fibrosis have been described.[91]

The peripheral vestibular system may also be involved during the second stage of infection, in which both the VIIIth cranial nerve and labyrinth are involved in fulminant meningoneurolabyrinthitis.

Clinical Presentation

The clinical course of syphilis has been divided into three stages. Primary syphilis typically is seen in the acquired form, and is characterized by the presence of a chancre (a painless, nonpurulent, and indurated ulcer in the region of sexual contact), which usually appears 3 weeks after initial infection. Although usually solitary, multiple ulcers may be seen in HIV-infected patients;[87] however chancres may go unnoticed and may only be seen in a third of cases.[92] Regional lymphadenopathy also may be present in primary syphilis. Symptoms last from 3 to 90 days, but often go unnoticed.[93]

Secondary syphilis occurs weeks after the chancre has healed, and is characterized by a variety of mucosal and cutaneous lesions that appear 2 to 12 weeks after initial infection (it may overlap the primary stage in up to 75% of HIV-infected patients), as well as the presence of constitutional symptoms such as fever and malaise. Asymptomatic meningitis may occur in up to 40% of patients[93] although associated sudden progressive bilateral hearing loss and vertigo are rare.[88] Other organ systems may be involved, including the liver, kidney, eyes, and joints. The latent phase follows, which is characterized by a lengthy period free of symptoms.

Tertiary syphilis, which is similar to late congenital syphilis, manifests years after initial infection. It is characterized by cardiovascular, gummatous, and neurologic involvement. Approximately 15 to 40% of untreated patients will progress to the third stage.[87]

Neurosyphilis is composed of meningovascular and parenchymal lesions. Chronic meningitis and vasculitis may involve the VIIIth cranial nerve. In addition, parenchymal diseases, including demyelination (tabes dorsalis), motor weakness, and sensory loss may adversely affect balance. Inner ear involvement during the tertiary phase may produce symptoms identical to those seen in Ménière's disease.[88,94] Left untreated, otogenic syphilis has a more aggressive course than Ménière's disease, commonly involving both ears and leading to profound deafness. Physical exam reveals signs consistent with sensorineural hearing loss and peripheral vestibular loss. Hennebert's sign (vertigo and nystagmus induced with air pressure to the middle ear) and Tullio's phenomenon (vertigo and nystagmus caused by loud noise) may be associated with tertiary syphilis.

Early congenital syphilis occurs during the first 2 years of life. Symptoms vary from asymptomatic to multiorgan involvement. Late manifestations of syphilis include the presence of hearing loss, interstitial keratitis, and notched incisors (Hutchinson's triad). The hearing loss is sudden and usually occurs around the age of 8 to 10.[93]

Investigations

The diagnosis of syphilis depends on clinical findings, histological examination of lesions, and serologic testing for syphilis. The Venereal Disease Research Laboratory (VDRL) screening test and rapid plasma reagin (RPR) are useful screening tests, but lack sufficient sensitivity for both early and late syphilis.[93] Treponemal tests, such as the fluorescent treponemal antibody absorption test (FTA-ABS) or a microhemagglutination test for *T. pallidum* (MHA-TP) have higher sensitivity and specificity, and are often required for diagnosis. In fact, routine serologic testing for otosyphilis is recommended in all cases of idiopathic progressive sensorineural hearing loss.[95] In addition, the diagnosis of neurosyphilis may require testing of CSF.[93] In order to be considered a confirmed case of congenital syphilis, *T. pallidum* must be identified within the tissues on histology.[96]

Treatment

Penicillin-based antibiotics (or an alternative if allergic) are the treatment of choice, with duration varied by stage of disease. The use of corticosteroids in the treatment of otogenic syphilis is controversial.[88,97–100]

Prognosis

The prognosis for hearing loss in otogenic syphilis is poor, with hearing improvement seen in less that one-third of treated patients.[89]

Labyrinthitis

Definition

Acute infection of the labyrinth by virus or bacteria can lead to symptoms of vertigo and hearing loss. It is important to realize that the term labyrinthitis is reserved for infections that result in both hearing loss and vestibular symptoms. Viral labyrinthitis occurs secondary to systemic viral infection, and is more common.[101] Bacterial labyrinthitis occurs as a complication of meningitis and otitis media.

Incidence and Epidemiology

Bacterial labyrinthitis secondary to meningitis accounts for up to one third of cases of postnatal acquired hearing loss.[102] Hearing loss occurs in approximately 10% of children with meningitis.[103,104] Bacterial meningitis is less common in the adult, and secondary labyrinthitis occurs less commonly in adult than child. Suppurative otitis media is a less common cause of labyrinthitis.[101,105,106]

Viral labyrinthitis may occur as part of a multisystemic viral infection (eg, rubella, measles, mumps, herpes zoster, CMV). In all of these cases, hearing loss is a much more common symptom of labyrinthine involvement than is vertigo. In the adult, sudden sensorineural hearing loss, which is most commonly viral in origin, occurs with an incidence of 1 per 10,000.[107] Forty percent of this patient group manifest vertigo or disequilibrium as well.[108]

Microbiology

Bacterial meningitis in the child is most commonly caused by *Streptococcus pneumoniae, Nesseria meningitides*, and *Haemophilus influenzae*.[109] The most common causes of bacterial meningitis in adults are due to *Streptococcus pneumonia* and *Nesseria meningitides*.[110]

Labyrinthitis secondary to acute otitis media is caused by *Streptococcus and*

Staphylococcus, although other organisms such as *H. influenzae* and *Moraxella catarrhalis* may be culprit.[101,111,112] When it occurs with secondary chronic otitis media due to cholesteatoma induced erosion of the labyrinth, *S. aureus* and gram negative organisms are more frequently encountered.[101] Concomitant positive viral serologies have been shown in patients with bacterial labyrinthitis; their significance is yet to be elucidated.[111] Rarely, fungi may invade the ear (eg, cryptococcus), typically in the face of systemic immune compromise.

Pathology

Acute labyrinthitis can be classified as serous or suppurative. Serous labyrinthitis is the result of inflammatory and toxic mediators. Suppurative labyrinthitis involves direct bacterial invasion of the otic capsule. Bacteria spreads to the labyrinth from the central nervous system through the internal auditory canal or the cochlear aqueduct. Bacterial infection causes an inflammatory infiltrate within the fluid compartments of the inner ear, with subsequent destruction of cellular constituents.[113] During the healing phase, fibrous tissue is then generated with subsequent osteoneogenesis. The consequence of viral infections are more variable, depending on the affinity of the infecting virus for particular cell types.

Clinical Presentation

Bacterial labyrinthitis presents with sudden hearing loss and vertigo lasting for days. The hearing loss usually is severe to profound and permanent. As the vertigo resolves, the patient is left with positional disequilibrium of variable duration characteristic of an uncompensated vestibular loss. In patients with meningitis, both the hearing loss and vertigo may be initially obscured owing to the overall clinical deterioration. In cases of bacterial labyrinthitis resulting from otitis media, physical exam demonstrates acute otitis media or presence of cholesteatoma. Tuning fork exams are consistent with a pure sensorineural hearing loss in cases resulting from bacterial meningitis, and a mixed hearing loss in cases due to otitis media. Nystagmus patterns are consistent with unilateral peripheral irritative, or more commonly a paretic lesion. Additional symptoms may include constitutional symptoms, nausea, vomiting, imbalance, and pain, diaphoresis, or pallor.

The presentation of viral labyrinthitis usually is less severe than bacterial labyrinthitis. It typically manifests as a sudden decline in hearing of variable degree and associated vertigo. The observation of vesicles, especially with otalgia, would be a reason to suspect Ramsey Hunt syndrome.

Investigations

Patients with meningitis require appropriate medical work-up typically including a lumbar puncture. CT scan is indicated in cases of chronic otitis media with cholesteatoma in order to evaluate the extent of disease and aid in surgical planning. Antibiotic coverage should be started immediately and should be culture directed. MRI is the most sensitive radiologic test for labyrinthitis and is useful for evaluating retrocochlear pathology as well. Audiometric evaluation is indicated in all cases of labyrinthitis to document the hearing loss. Vestibular testing may be obtained when the patient is stable.

Treatment

Bacterial labyrinthitis secondary to meningitis is treated with parenteral antibiotic and corticosteroids. Studies indicate that corticosteroids given prophylactically at the time of diagnosis of acute bacterial meningitis decrease the incidence of severe hearing loss as well as the pathologic changes of labyrinthitis ossificans.[114,115]

Labyrinthitis secondary to acute otitis media is treated with parenteral antibiotics, corticosteroids, and myringotomy with drainage of the ear and tube placement.[105] Labyrinthitis secondary to chronic otitis media with cholesteotoma requires similar drug therapy, as well as mastoidectomy to remove disease. Viral labyrinthitis is treated with high-dose corticosteroids. Antiviral therapy is usually considered empirically in suspected cases of viral labyrinthitis, although there is no clear evidence of its efficacy in preventing or improving hearing loss.[116]

Prognosis

Bacterial infections of the inner ear carry a very poor prognosis for preservation of inner ear function. Labyrinthitis ossificans is due to fibrous or bony replacement of the labyrinth; it most commonly results from acute labyrinthitis arising due to bacterial meningitis. There is evidence to suggest that steroids can prevent this progression.[115] In viral infection, the prognosis for recovery of at least some hearing is better than that seen in bacterial infection.

Ototoxicity

Definition

A variety of chemicals cause damage to the inner ear. Most agents are toxic only to the cochlea. A noted exception is the commonly used aminoglycoside antibiotics, which are major vestibulotoxins.

Incidence and Epidemiology

Good prospective data concerning the incidence of aminoglycoside ototoxicity are not available. Individual susceptibility to aminoglycosides is highly variable. Factors that predispose to ototoxicity include renal failure, advanced age, concurrent use of other ototoxic agents, family history of susceptibility, and pre-existing sensorineural hearing loss.[117] In general, systemically administered aminoglycosides are more toxic than topical administration (ie, eardrops). Variations in individual susceptibility to aminoglycosides may be mediated by a mutation in mitochondrial DNA.[118,119]

Pathology

The dose limiting side effects of the aminoglycoside antibiotics are ototoxicity and nephrotoxicity; each effect is independent of the other.[120] Gentamicin and streptomycin are the two aminoglycosides with the greatest vestibulotoxicity, with tobramycin also having significant vestibular potential.[121] Hair cells in the cochlea (OHC>IHC) and the vestibule (Type I > Type II) demonstrate degeneration when exposed to aminoglycosides. The basal regions of the cochlea, the apices of the cristae, and the striolar region of the maculae are the regions most susceptible to damage. More recent data suggest that spiral ganglion cells may be injured directly, in addition to hair cells.[122] In addition, the fluid and electrolyte regulating stria vascularis of the cochlea and dark cells of the vestibule also demonstrate edema and degeneration when exposed to aminoglycosides.

The biochemical mechanisms by which aminoglycosides exert these ototoxic effects are too complex to be fully elucidated in this discussion. Current concepts include the metabolism of aminoglycosides in the liver, during which time they are bound to iron.[123] The aminoglycoside-iron complex then generates reactive oxygen species in the inner ear, which induces oxidative damage.

Clinical Presentation

Aminoglycoside ototoxicity manifests as an acute onset of bilateral, high frequency sensorineural hearing loss (the lower frequencies may be involved as well). The hearing loss is usually permanent. On the other hand, patients may present with symptoms of bilateral vestibular hypofunction, such as disequilibrium or imbalance with oscillopsia; frank vertigo is not typical. In general, vestibular dysfunction occurs without accompanying injury to the auditory system, and patients may compensate well with vestibular rehabilitation.[120,124] Symptoms may manifest as soon as four hours after initial treatment, although some patient may not be affected until weeks after treatment cessation.[120] In patients who are severely debilitated during the period of antibiotic administration, the immediate effects may not be apparent, and may manifest later as hearing loss or disequilibrium.

Investigations

Audiometry reveals sensorineural hearing loss and vestibular testing shows bilateral vestibular hypofunction.

Treatment

Hearing aid amplification and vestibular rehabilitation are the mainstays of treatment. A variety of measures have been advocated to prevent aminoglycoside ototoxicity, including monitoring of drug levels, consideration of renal function with regards to dosing, and avoidance of other ototoxic medications. Unfortunately, because of the variation in an individual's susceptibility, these measures cannot prevent all cases of ototoxicity and no dose of aminoglycosides should be considered a completely safe dose. Animal studies have shown that hair cells can be protected from aminoglycoside induced damage, especially with the use of antioxidants and iron-chelators; however, there are no otoprotective medications available to humans.[120,123]

Prognosis

Bilateral vestibular hypofunction can very disabling, yet many patients adapt well to the loss, particularly when rehabilitation regimens are initiated.[109]

Immunologic—Autoimmune Inner Ear Disease

Definition

Autoimmune inner ear disease (AIED) was first described by McCabe in 1979.[126] The patient's own immune system may become reactive to self-antigen resulting in autoimmune disease. Autoimmune inner ear disease may be associated with systemic disease or may occur as an organ specific process.[126–129]

Incidence and Epidemiology

Autoimmune inner ear disease is a rare cause of hearing loss and dizziness accounting for less than 1% of all cases.[130] Inner ear dysfunction is a rare complication of multisystem autoimmune disease.[127,131] Similarly, primary autoimmune inner ear disease represents a rare cause of labyrinthine pathology. However, AIED is potentially reversible, and must be considered in the appropriate clinical setting.

Pathology

Target sites within the inner ear for autoimmune reactions may include its cellular constituents and the vascular supply. A variety of disorders characterized by vasculitis are known to result in labyrinthine pathology. In addition, animal models have demonstrated the inner ear's ability to mount an immune response, manifested by an inflammatory cellular infiltrate within the scalae.[132] Analysis of temporal bones derived from animals with experimental labyrinthitis and humans who have suffered labyrinthine pathology secondary to systemic autoimmune disease reveal similar findings.[113,133] These include degeneration of the organ of Corti, vestibular sensory organs, stria vascularis, and dark cell layers, as well as fibrosis and osteoneogenesis.

Clinical Presentation

Autoimmune inner era disease presents as a rapidly progressive (over weeks to months), asymmetric, hearing loss.[126] Hearing levels may fluctuate during the acute phases of the disease. Hearing loss is frequently bilateral, occurring in approximately 80% of patients.[134] A hallmark of the hearing loss is that it improves with corticosteroid administration. Vestibular complaints, most commonly vertigo, are present in a majority of patients.[129,134] Tinnitus and aural fullness are commonly present as well. The initial presentation of AIED may be difficult to differentiate from Ménière's disease; they are distinguished by AIED's more aggressive course, as well as its higher incidence of bilateral involvement. Although some authors report a female predilection,[130] this has not been seen in every series.[134]

Investigations

There are no specific tests for AIED. Serial audiometric evaluations provide critical data to the rate and degree of hearing loss. Vestibular testing reveals evidence of a peripheral vestibular injury. As some 30% of patients with primary AIED present with systemic autoimmune disease, an immune profile is indicated. This should include a complete blood cell count, erythrocyte sedimentation rate, electrolytes, blood urea nitrogen, creatinine, urinalysis, antinuclear antibodies, rheumatoid factor, complement levels, FTA-ABS, smooth muscle antibody, TSH, anti-microsomal antibodies, and anti-gliadin antibodies (for celiac diseases). Lyme titers may be indicated in endemic areas. Tests for HIV and diabetes may be indicated as well, given their association with autoimmune disease.[130] An MRI is required to rule-out retrocochlear pathology and demyelinating diseases.

Several tests have been advocated as being useful in the diagnosis of organ specific AIED. Tests of cellular immunity, including the lymphocyte migration inhibition assay and the lymphocyte transformation test have been advocated by several authors; however, their accuracy has not been validated.[126,135] Circulating antibody to a 68- to 72-kilodalton protein is suggested by some to be a marker for AIED, as well as a marker of steroid-responsiveness; however, there is no clear evidence to suggest that it is specific for AIED[136–138] (although there is some recent data supporting that serum antibodies to inner ear supporting cells in fact may predict steroid-responsiveness.[139]). Ultimately, the diagnosis of AIED rests on a positive response to a trial of immunosuppression (steroids).

Treatment

Patients with suspected AIED should be treated with a one month course of steroids (1–2 mg/kg/day), followed by a slow taper. Steroids should be started as soon as the diagnosis is suspected since the hearing loss can progress and become irreversible over a relative short period of time (weeks to months). Patients are then maintained on a maintenance dose of 10 to 20 mg of prednisone either daily or every other day; if symptoms worsen or recur, another course of high dose steroids is initiated.[130] Although traditionally used to maintain the hearing benefit achieved with steroids, methotrexate is no longer indicated and has been shown to be ineffective in maintaining hearing improvement.[140] Cyclophosphamide has also been suggested as a treatment option either alone in steroid-resistant patients or in conjunction with or following steroids[126,141]; however, the precise role of cyclophosphamide in AIED has not been clearly defined.

Prognosis

Untreated, patients are at risk of developing profound bilateral sensorineural hearing loss, as well as significant vestibular dysfunction. A majority of patients respond to steroids, although some patients are steroid-unresponsive, and continue to have a decline in their hearing. Even in steroid-responsive patients, management can be challenging as hearing loss may progress upon cessation of steroids. A multidisciplinary approach combining the expertise of an otolaryngologist with a rheumatologist or immunologist is necessary. In patients in whom long-term immunosuppression poses too great a risk, or in patients resistant to immunosuppression, cochlear implantation is a viable alternative.

References

1. Universal Screening for Hearing Loss in Newborns. U.S. Preventive Services Task Force Recommendation Statement. *Pediatrics.* 2008;122(1):143.

2. Year 2000 Position Statement: principles and guidelines for early hearing detection and intervention programs. *Pediatrics.* 2000;106(4):798.
3. Steel K, Bock GR. Hereditary inner-ear abnormalities in animals: relationships with human abnormalities. *Arch Otolaryngol.* 1983;109(1):22–29.
4. Grundfast KM. Syndromic hereditary hearing impairment. In: Lalwani AK, Grundfast KM, eds. *Pediatric Otology and Neurotology.* Philadelphia, PA: Lippincott Raven; 1998, 341–364.
5. Chan KH, Eelkema EA, Furman JM, Kamerer DB. Familial sensorineural hearing loss: a correlative study of audiologic, radiologic, and vestibular findings. *Ann Otol Rhinol Laryngol.* 1991;100:620–625.
6. Griffith AJ, Telian SA, Downs C, et al. Familial Mondini dysplasia. *Laryngoscope.* 1998;108(9):1368–1373.
7. Irving RM, H.T., Moffat DA, et al. Somatic neurofibromatosis type 2 gene mutations and growth characteristics in vestibular schwannoma. *Am J Otol.* 1997;18(6):754–760.
8. Jackler RK, House WF. Congenital malformations of the inner ear: a classification based on embryogenesis. *Laryngoscope.* 1987;97(3 pt 2 suppl 40): 2–14.
9. Angeli S. Value of vestibular testing in young children with sensorineural hearing loss. *Arch Otolaryngol Head Neck Surg.* 2003;129(4):478–482.
10. Robson CD. Congenital hearing impairment. *Pediatr Radiol.* 2006;36(4): 309–324.
11. Telian, SA. Comments about the value of vestibular testing in young children with sensorineural hearing loss. *Arch Otolaryngol Head Neck Surg.* 2003; 129(4):483–484.
12. Goebel JA. Should we screen hearing-impaired children for vestibular dysfunction? *Arch Otolaryngol Head Neck Surg.* 2003;129(4):482–483.
13. Kaga K. Vestibular compensation in infants and children with congenital and acquired vestibular loss in both ears. *Int J Pediatr Otorhinolaryngol.* 1999; 49(3):215.
14. Hasso AN, Ledington JA. Traumatic injuries of the temporal bone. *Otolaryngol Clin North Am.* 1988;21:295–316.
15. Cannon CR, Jahrsdoerfer RA. Temporal bine fractures: review of 90 cases. *Arch Otolaryngol.* 1983;109(5):285–288.
16. Johnson F, Semaan MT, Megerian CA. Temporal bone fractures: evaluation and management in the modern era. *Otolaryngol Clin North Am.* 2008;41(3): 597–618.
17. Dahiya R, Keller JD, Litofsky NS, Bankey PE, Bonassar LJ, Megerian CA. Temporal bone fractures: otic capsule sparing versus otic capsule violating clinical and radiographic considerations. *J Trauma.* 1999;47(6):1079–1083.
18. Little SC, Kesser BW. Radiographic classification of temporal bone fractures: clinical predictability using a new system. *Arch Otolaryngol Head Neck Surg.* 2006;132(12):1300–1304.
19. Schuknecht B, Graetz K. Radiologic assessment of maxillofacial, mandibular, and skull base trauma. *Eur Radiol.* 2005;15(3):560–568.
20. Camilleri AE, Toner JG, Howarth KL, Hampton S, Ramsden RT. Cochlear implantation following temporal bone fracture. *J Laryngol Otol.* 1999;113(5): 454–457.
21. Bird J, Humphriss RL, Prevost AT. The evidence base for the application of contralateral bone anchored hearing aids in acquired unilateral sensorineural hearing loss in adults. *Clin Otolaryngol.* 2006;31(1):6–14.
22. Cantais E, Louge P, Suppini A, Foster PP, Palmier B. Right-to-left shunt and risk of decompression illness with cochleovestibular and cerebral symptoms in divers: case control study in 101 consecutive dive accidents. *Crit Care Med.* 2003;31(1):84–88.
23. Klingmann C, Praetorius M, Baumann I, Plinkert PK. Barotrauma and decompression illness of the inner ear: 46 cases

during treatment and follow-up. *Otol Neurotol.* 2007;28(4):447–454.

24. Wicks RE. Alternobaric vertigo: an aeromedical review. *Aviat Space Environ Med.* 1989;60(1):67–72.
25. Parell GJ, Becker GD. Conservative management of inner ear barotrauma resulting from scuba diving. *Otolaryngol Head Neck Surg.* 1985;93(3):393–397.
26. Farmer JC, Thomas WG, Youngblood DG, Bennett PB. Inner ear decompression sickness. *Laryngoscope.* 1976;86(9): 1315–1327.
27. Schuknecht HF, Witt RL. Suppressed sneezing as a cause of hearing loss and vertigo. *Am J Otolaryngol.* 1985;6(6): 468–470.
28. Farmer J. Diving injuries of the inner ear. *Ann Otol Rhinol Laryngol.* 1977; 86(suppl):1–20.
29. Phelps PD. Congenital cerebrospinal fluid fistulae of the petrous temporal bone. *Clin Otolaryngol Allied Sci.* 1986; 11(2):79–92.
30. Emmet JR, Shea JJ. Traumatic perilymph fistula. *Laryngoscope.* 1980;90(9): 1512–1520.
31. Maitland CG. Perilymphatic fistula. *Curr Neurol Neurosci Rep.* 2001;1(5): 486–491.
32. Goodhill V. Sudden deafness and round window rupture. *Laryngoscope.* 1971;81(9):1462–1474.
33. Shea JJ. The myth of spontaneous perilymph fistula. *Otolaryngol Head Neck Surg.* 1992;107(5):613–616.
34. Friedland DR, Wackym PA. A critical appraisal of spontaneous perilymphatic fistulas of the inner ear [erratum appears in *Am J Otol.* 1999 Jul;20(4):560]. *Am J Otol.* 1999;20(2):261–276; discussion 276–279.
35. Rizer FM, House JW. Perilymph fistulas: the House Ear Clinic experience. *Otolaryngol Head Neck Surg.* 1991; 104(2):239–243.
36. Vartiainen E, Nuutinen J, Karjalainen S, Nykänen K. Perilymph fistula—a diagnostic dilemma. *J Laryngol Otol.* 1991;105(4):270–273.
37. Buchman CA, Luxford WM, Hirsch BE, Fucci MJ, Kelly RH. Beta-2 transferrin assay in the identification of perilymph. *Am J Otol.* 1999;20(2): 174–178.
38. Rauch SD. Transferrin microheterogeneity in human perilymph. *Laryngoscope.* 2000;110(4):545–552.
39. Poe DS, Rebeiz EE, Pankratov MM. Evaluation of perilymphatic fistulas by middle ear endoscopy. *Am J Otol.* 1992;13(6):529–533.
40. Poe DS, Bottrill ID. Comparison of endoscopic and surgical explorations for perilymphatic fistulas. *Am J Otol.* 1994;15(6):735–738.
41. Tato JM, Tato JM Jr. Otosclerosis and races. *Ann Otol Rhinol Laryngol.* 1967; 76(5):1018–1025.
42. Altmann FA, Glasgold A, Macduff JP. The incidence of otosclerosis as related to race and sex. *Ann Otol Rhinol Laryngol.* 1967;76(2):377–392.
43. Moumoulidis I, Axon P, Baguley D, Reid E. A review on the genetics of otosclerosis. *Clin Otolaryngol.* 2007; 32(4):239–247.
44. Morrison AW. Genetic factors in otosclerosis. *Ann R Coll Surg Engl.* 1967; 41(2):202–237.
45. Thys M, Van Den Bogaert K, Iliadou V, et al. A seventh locus for otosclerosis, OTSC7, maps to chromosome 6q13-16.1. *Euro J Hum Gen.* 2007;15(3): 362–368.
46. Bel Hadj Ali I, Thys M, Beltaief N, et al. A new locus for otosclerosis, OTSC8, maps to the pericentromeric region of chromosome 9. *Hum Gen.* 2008;123(3): 267–272.
47. McKenna MJ, Kristiansen AG, Bartley ML, Rogus JJ, Haines JL. Association of COL1A1 and otosclerosis: evidence for a shared genetic etiology with mild osteogenesis imperfecta. *Am J Otol.* 1998;19(5):604–610.

48. McKenna MJ, Kristiansen AG, Haines J. Polymerase chain reaction amplification of a measles virus sequence from human temporal bone sections with active otosclerosis. *Am J Otol.* 1996;17(6):827–830.
49. Chen W, Meyer NC, McKenna MJ, et al. Single-nucleotide polymorphisms in the COL1A1 regulatory regions are associated with otosclerosis. *Clin Gen.* 2007;71(5):406–414.
50. Schuknecht H. Pathology of the Ear. In: *Pathology of the Ear.* Philadelphia, PA: Lea & Febinger; 1993:249–254, 366–378.
51. Kwok OT, Nadol JB Jr. Correlation of otosclerotic foci and degenerative changes in the organ of Corti and spiral ganglion. *Am J Otolaryngol.* 1989; 10(1):1–12.
52. Saim L, Nadol JB Jr. Vestibular symptoms in otosclerosis—correlation of otosclerotic involvement of vestibular apparatus and Scarpa's ganglion cell count. *Am J Otol.* 1996;17(2):263–270.
53. Paparella MM, Mancini F, Liston SL. Otosclerosis and ménière's syndrome: diagnosis and treatment. *Laryngoscope.* 1984;94(11 pt 1):1414–1417.
54. McCabe BF. Otosclerosis and vertigo. *Trans Pac Coast Otoophthalmol Soc Annu Meet.* 1966;47:37–42.
55. Ghorayeb BY, Linthicum FH Jr. Otosclerotic inner ear syndrome. *Ann Otol Rhinol Laryngol.* 1978;87(1 pt 1):85–90.
56. Merchant SN, Rosowski JJ, McKenna MJ. Superior semicircular canal dehiscence mimicking otosclerotic hearing loss. *Adv Oto-Rhino-Laryngol.* 2007;65: 137–145.
57. Minor LB, Carey JP, Cremer PD, Lustig LR, Streubel SO, Ruckenstein MJ. Dehiscence of bone overlying the superior canal as a cause of apparent conductive hearing loss. *Otol Neurotol.* 2003;24(2):270–278.
58. Hansen MC. Otosclerosis and sensorineural hearing loss. A clinical study. *Arch Otolaryngol.* 1983;109(9):598–600.
59. Cody DT, Baker HL Jr. Otosclerosis: vestibular symptoms and sensorineural hearing loss. *Ann Otol Rhinol Laryngol.* 1978;87(6 pt 1):778–796.
60. Ruckenstein MJ, Rafter KO, Montes M, Bigelow DC. Management of far advanced otosclerosis in the era of cochlear implantation. *Otol Neurotol.* 2001;22(4):471–474.
61. Causse JR, Causse JB, Uriel J, Berges J, Shambaugh GE Jr, Bretlau P. Sodium fluoride therapy. *Am J Otol.* 1993;14(5): 482–490.
62. Tos M, Stangerup SE, Cayé-Thomasen P, Tos T, Thomsen J. What is the real incidence of vestibular schwannoma? *Arch Otolaryngol Head Neck Surg.* 2004;130(2):216–220.
63. Nestor JJ, Korol HW, Nutik SL, Smith R. The incidence of acoustic neuromas. *Arch Otolaryngol Head Neck Surg.* 1988;114(6):680.
64. Lanser MJ, Sussman SA, Frazer K. Epidemiology, pathogenesis, and genetics of acoustic tumors. *Otolaryngol Clin North Am.* 1992;25(3):499–520.
65. Anderson TD, Loevner LA, Bigelow DC, Mirza N. Prevalence of unsuspected acoustic neuroma found by magnetic resonance imaging. *Otolaryngol Head Neck Surg.* 2000;122(5): 643–646.
66. Sekhar LN, Jannetta PJ. Cerebellopontine angle meningiomas. Microsurgical excision and follow-up results. *J Neurosurg.* 1984;60(3):500–505.
67. Jackler RK, Parker DA. Radiographic differential diagnosis of petrous apex lesions. *Am J Otol.* 1992;13(6):561–574.
68. Sterkers JM, Perre J, Viala P, Foncin JF. The origin of acoustic neuromas. *Acta Oto-Laryngologica.* 1987;103(5–6): 427–431.
69. Moffat DA, Irving RM. The molecular genetics of vestibular schwannoma. *J Laryngol Otol.* 1995;109(5):381–384.
70. Bikhazi PH, Lalwani AK, Kim EJ, et al. Germline screening of the NF-2 gene

in families with unilateral vestibular schwannoma. *Otolaryngol Head Neck Surg.* 1998;119(1):1–6.

71. Neff BA, Welling DB, Akhmametyeva E, Chang LS. The molecular biology of vestibular schwannomas: dissecting the pathogenic process at the molecular level. *Otol Neurotol.* 2006;27(2):197–208.
72. Langford LA. Pathology of meningiomas. *J Neuro-Oncol.* 1996;29(3):217–221.
73. Jackler RK, Cho M. A new theory to explain the genesis of petrous apex cholesterol granuloma. *Otol Neurotol.* 2003;24:96–106.
74. Pyle GM, Wiet RJ. Petrous apex cholesteatoma: exteriorization vs. subtotal petrosectomy with obliteration. *Skull Base Surg.* 1991;1(2):97–104.
75. van Leeuwen JP, Cremers CW, Thewissen NP, Harhangi BS, Meijer E. Acoustic neuroma: correlation among tumor size, symptoms, and patient age. *Laryngoscope.* 1995;105(7):701–707.
76. Selesnick SH, Jackler RK, Pitts LW. The changing clinical presentation of acoustic tumors in the MRI era. *Laryngoscope.* 1993;103(4 pt 1):431–436.
77. Selesnick SH, Jackler RK. Clinical manifestations and audiologic diagnosis of acoustic neuromas. *Otolaryngol Clin North Am.* 1992;25(3):521–551.
78. Laird FJ, Harner SG, Laws ER Jr, Reese DF. Meningiomas of the cerebellopontine angle. *Otolaryngol Head Neck Surg.* 1985;93(2):163–167.
79. Baguley DM, Beynon GJ, Grey PL, Hardy DG, Moffat DA. Audio-vestibular findings in meningioma of the cerebellopontine angle: a retrospective review. *J Laryngol Otol.* 1997;111(11):1022–1026.
80. Thedinger BA, Nadol JB Jr, Montgomery WW, Thedinger BS, Greenberg JJ. Radiographic diagnosis, surgical treatment, and long-term follow-up of cholesterol granulomas of the petrous apex. *Laryngoscope.* 1989;99(9):896–907.
81. Goldofsky E, Hoffman RA, Holliday RA, Cohen NL. Cholesterol cysts of the temporal bone: diagnosis and treatment. *Ann Otol Rhinol Laryngol.* 1991;100(3):181–187.
82. Shelton C, Harnsberger HR, Allen R, King B. Fast spin echo magnetic resonance imaging: clinical application in screening for acoustic neuroma. *Otolaryngol Head Neck Surg.* 1996;114(1):71–76.
83. Linker SP, Ruckenstein MJ, Acker J, Gardner G. An accurate, cost-effective approach for diagnosing retrocochlear lesions utilizing the T2-weighted, fast-spin echo magnetic resonance imaging scan. *Laryngoscope.* 1997;107(11 pt 1):1525–1529.
84. Doyle KJ. Is there still a role for auditory brainstem response audiometry in the diagnosis of acoustic neuroma? *Arch Otolaryngol Head Neck Surg.* 1999;125(2):232–234.
85. Abram S, Rosenblatt P, Holcomb S. Stereotactic radiation techniques in the treatment of acoustic schwannomas. *Otolaryngologic Clin North Am.* 2008;40(3):571–588.
86. Giddings NA, Brackmann DE, Kwartler JA. Transcanal infracochlear approach to the petrous apex. *Otolaryngol Head Neck Surg.* 1991;104(1):29–36.
87. Zetola NM, Engelman J, Jensen TP, Klausner JD. Syphilis in the United States: an update for clinicians with an emphasis on HIV coinfection [erratum appears in *Mayo Clin Proc.* 2007;82(11):1434]. *Mayo Clin Proc.* 2007;82(9):1091–1102.
88. Darmstadt GL, Harris JP. Luetic hearing loss: clinical presentation, diagnosis, and treatment. *Am J Otolaryngol.* 1989;10(6):410–421.
89. Yimtae K, Srirompotong S, Lertsukprasert K. Otosyphilis: a review of 85 cases. *Otolaryngol Head Neck Surg.* 2007;136(1):67–71.
90. Allam AF. Pathology of the human spiral ligament. *J Laryngol Otol.* 1970;84(8):765–779.

91. Belal A Jr, Linthicum FH Jr. Pathology of congenital syphilitic labyrinthitis. *Am J Otolaryngol.* 1980;1(2):109–118.
92. DiCarlo RP, Martin DH. The clinical diagnosis of genital ulcer disease in men. *Clin Infect Dis.* 1997;25(2):292–298.
93. Singh AE, Romanowski B. Syphilis: review with emphasis on clinical, epidemiologic, and some biologic features. *Clin Microbiol Rev.* 1999;12(2): 187–209.
94. Steckelberg JM, McDonald TJ. Otologic involvement in late syphilis. *Laryngoscope.* 1984;94(6):753–757.
95. Abuzeid WM, Ruckenstein MJ. Spirochetes in otology: are we testing for the right pathogens? *Otolaryngol Head Neck Surg.* 2008;138(1):107–109.
96. Centers for Disease (CDC). Syphilis and congenital syphilis—United States, 1985–1988. *MMWR Morb Mortal Wkly Rep.* 1988;37(32):486–489.
97. Linstrom CJ, Gleich LL. Otosyphilis: diagnostic and therapeutic update. *J Otolaryngol.* 1993;22(6):401–408.
98. Dobbin JM, Perkins JH. Otosyphilis and hearing loss: response to penicillin and steroid therapy. *Laryngoscope.* 1983;93(12):1540–1543.
99. Chan YM, Adams DA, Kerr AG. Syphilitic labyrinthitis—an update. *J Laryngol Otol.* 1995;109(8):719–725.
100. Zoller M, Wilson WR, Nadol JB Jr. Treatment of syphilitic hearing loss. Combined penicillin and steroid therapy in 29 patients. *Ann Otol Rhinol Laryngol.* 1979;88(2 pt 1):160–165.
101. Kitsko DJ, Dohar JE. Inner ear and facial nerve complications of acute otitis media, including vertigo. *Curr Allergy Asthma Rep.* 2007;7(6):444–450.
102. Das VK. Aetiology of bilateral sensorineural hearing impairment in children: a 10 year study. *Arch Dis Child.* 1996;74(1):8–12.
103. Richardson MP, Reid A, Tarlow MJ, Rudd PT. Hearing loss during bacterial meningitis [erratum appears in *Arch Dis Child.* 1997;76(4):386]. *Arch Dis Child.* 1997;76(2):134–138.
104. Fortnum HM. Hearing impairment after bacterial meningitis: a review. *Arch Dis Child.* 1992;67(9):1128–1133.
105. Goldstein NA, Casselbrant ML, Bluestone CD, Kurs-Lasky M. Intratemporal complications of acute otitis media in infants and children. *Otolaryngol Head Neck Surg.* 1998;119(5):444–454.
106. Albers FW. Complications of otitis media: the importance of early recognition. *Am J Otol.* 1999;20(1):9–12.
107. Byl FM. Seventy-six cases of presumed sudden hearing loss occurring in 1973: prognosis and incidence. *Laryngoscope.* 1977;87(5 pt 1):817–825.
108. Shaia FT, Sheehy JL. Sudden sensorineural hearing impairment: a report of 1,220 cases. *Laryngoscope.* 1976;86(3): 389–398.
109. Tebruegge M, Curtis N. Epidemiology, etiology, pathogenesis, and diagnosis of recurrent bacterial meningitis. *Clin Microbiol Rev.* 2008;21(3):519–537.
110. Durand ML, Calderwood SB, Weber DJ, et al. Acute bacterial meningitis in adults—a review of 493 episodes. *N Engl J Med.* 1993;328(1):21–28.
111. Hydén D, Akerlind B, Peebo M. Inner ear and facial nerve complications of acute otitis media with focus on bacteriology and virology. *Acta Oto-Laryngologica.* 2006;126(5):460–466.
112. Block SL. Causative pathogens, antibiotic resistance and therapeutic considerations in acute otitis media. *Ped Infect Dis J.* 1997;16(4):449–456.
113. Merchant SN, Gopen Q. A human temporal bone study of acute bacterial meningogenic labyrinthitis. *Am J Otol.* 1996;17(3):375–385.
114. van de Beek D, de Gans J, McIntyre P, Prasad K. Corticosteroids for acute bacterial meningitis [update of *Cochrane Database Syst Rev.* 2003;(3):CD004405; PMID:12918010]. *Cochrane Database Syst Rev.* 2007;1:CD004405.

115. Hartnick CJ, Kim HH, Chute PM, Parisier SC. Preventing labyrinthitis ossificans: the role of steroids [erratum appears in *Arch Otolaryngol Head Neck Surg*. 2005;131(7):582. [Note: Kim HY corrected to Kim HH]. *Arch Otolaryngol Head Neck Surg*. 2001;127(2):180–183.
116. Westerlaken BO, Stokroos RJ, Dhooge IJ, Wit HP, Albers FW. Treatment of idiopathic sudden sensorineural hearing loss with antiviral therapy: a prospective, randomized, double-blind clinical trial. *Ann Otol Rhinol Laryngol.* 2003;112(11):993–1000.
117. Matz GJ. Aminoglycoside cochlear ototoxicity. *Otolaryngologic Clin North Am.* 1993;26(5):705–712.
118. Ensink RJ, Camp GV, Cremers CW. Mitochondrial inherited hearing loss. *Clin Otolaryngol Allied Sci.* 1998;23(1): 3–8.
119. Braverman I, Jaber L, Levi H, et al. Audiovestibular findings in patients with deafness caused by a mitochondrial susceptibility mutation and precipitated by an inherited nuclear mutation or aminoglycosides. *Arch Otolaryngol Head Neck Surg.* 1996; 122(9):1001–1004.
120. Guthrie OW. Aminoglycoside induced ototoxicity. *Toxicology.* 2008;249(2–3): 91–96.
121. Chiodo AA, Alberti PW. Experimental, clinical and preventive aspects of ototoxicity. *Euro Arch Oto-Rhino-Laryngol.* 1994;251(7):375–392.
122. Hinojosa R, Nelson EG, Lerner SA, Redleaf MI, Schramm DR. Aminoglycoside ototoxicity: a human temporal bone study. *Laryngoscope.* 2001;111(10): 1797–1805.
123. Schacht J. Aminoglycoside ototoxicity: prevention in sight? *Otolaryngol Head Neck Surg.* 1998;118(5):674–677.
124. Minor LB. Gentamicin-induced bilateral vestibular hypofunction. *JAMA.* 1998;279(7):541–544.
125. Telian SA, Shepard NT. Update on vestibular rehabilitation therapy. *Otolaryngologic Clin North Am.* 1996;29(2): 359–371.
126. McCabe BF. Autoimmune sensorineural hearing loss. *Ann Otol Rhinol Laryngol.* 1979;88(5 pt 1):585–589.
127. Schuknecht HF. Ear pathology in autoimmune disease. *Adv Oto-Rhino-Laryngol.* 1991;46:50–70.
128. Ruckenstein MJ, Harrison RV. Cochlear pathophysiology in Ménière's Disease—a critical appraisal. In: Harris J, ed. *Ménière's Disease.* The Hague, The Netherlands: Kugler; 1999:155–162.
129. Harris J, Ryan AF. Fundamental immune mechanisms of the brain and inner ear. *Otolaryngol Head Neck Surg.* 1995;112(6):639–653.
130. Bovo R, Aimoni C, Martini A. Immune-mediated inner ear disease. *Acta Oto-Laryngologica.* 2006;126(10):1012–1021.
131. Stephens SD, Luxon L, Hinchcliffe R. Immunological disorders and auditory lesions. *Audiology.* 1982;21(2): 128–148.
132. Harris JP, Fukuda S, Keithley EM. Spiral modiolar vein: its importance in inner ear inflammation. *Acta Oto-Laryngologica.* 1990;110(5–6):357–365.
133. Harris JP, Heydt J, Keithley EM, Chen MC. Immunopathology of the inner ear: an update. *Ann New York Acad Sci.* 1997;830:166–178.
134. Broughton SS, Meyerhoff WE, Cohen SB. Immune-mediated inner ear disease: 10-year experience. *Semin Arthritis Rheum.* 2004;34(2):544.
135. Hughes GB, Moscicki R, Barna BP, San Martin JE. Laboratory diagnosis of immune inner ear disease. *Am J Otol.* 1994;15(2):198–202.
136. Moscicki RA, San Martin JE, Quintero CH, Rauch SD, Nadol JB Jr, Bloch KJ. Serum antibody to inner ear proteins in patients with progressive hearing loss. Correlation with disease activity and response to corticosteroid treatment. *JAMA.* 1994;272(8):611–616.
137. Gottschlich S, Billings PB, Keithley EM, Weisman MH, Harris JP. Assessment

of serum antibodies in patients with rapidly progressive sensorineural hearing loss and Ménière's disease. *Laryngoscope.* 1995;105(12 pt 1):1347–1352.
138. Yeom K, Gray J, Nair TS, et al. Antibodies to HSP-70 in normal donors and autoimmune hearing loss patients. *Laryngoscope.* 2003;113(10):1770–1776.
139. Zeitoun H, Beckman JG, Arts HA, et al. Corticosteroid response and supporting cell antibody in autoimmune hearing loss. *Arch Otolaryngol Head Neck Surg.* 2005;131(8):665–672.
140. Harris JP, Weisman MH, Derebery JM, et al. Treatment of corticosteroid-responsive autoimmune inner ear disease with methotrexate: a randomized controlled trial. *JAMA.* 2003;290(14):1875–1883.
141. Rauch SD. Clinical management of immune-mediated inner-ear disease. *Ann N Y Acad Sci.* 1997;830:203–210.

7

Audiometric Testing

Michael J. Ruckenstein, MD

Pure-Tone Audiometry

Sensorineural hearing loss is one of the three required symptoms necessary for the diagnosis of Ménière's disease. As such, much attention has been focused on the configuration of the pure-tone audiogram, both at the time of the initial presentation, and as the disorder progresses.

In contrast to many other etiologies of sensorineural hearing loss (eg, ototoxicity, noise, aging), patients with Ménière's disease typically present with a low frequency hearing loss. Barber noted that, at the time of initial presentation, patients typically presented either with an isolated low-frequency hearing loss or a low and high-frequency loss with preservation of hearing in the mid-frequencies (inverted "V" pattern).[1] These observations were echoed by Stahle and colleagues, who reported that at the time of initial presentation, 28% of patients demonstrated an inverted "V" pure-tone audiogram, 20% of patients had an isolated low-frequency hearing loss, and 21% of patients had an isolated hearing loss (Fig 7–1).[2] Katsarkis examined audiometric data from a large series of patients with Ménière's disease, many of whom were followed for over 10 years, none of whom had undergone surgical treatment for this disorder.[3] These data indicate that, on average, the magnitude of low-frequency hearing loss was greater than that of high frequency hearing loss at the time of initial presentation.

As the disorder progresses, so does the hearing loss. In the majority of patients, the audiogram assumes a flat configuration, and the hearing ceases to fluctuate.[1,3] Katsarkis's data indicate that the low-frequency component of the hearing loss does slightly exceed the magnitude of the high-frequency loss.[3] Long-term follow-up studies indicate that the hearing levels begin to stabilize approximately 5 years after the onset of symptoms. A permanent threshold shift of approximately 50 dB has been noted in several studies,[3,4] although Katsarkis notes hearing loss levels to be of slightly

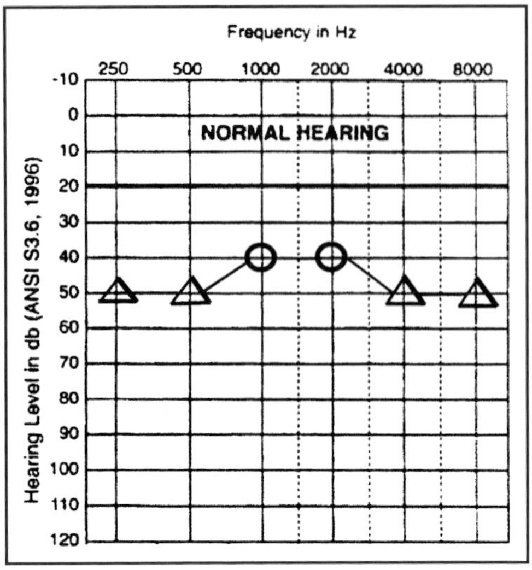

A

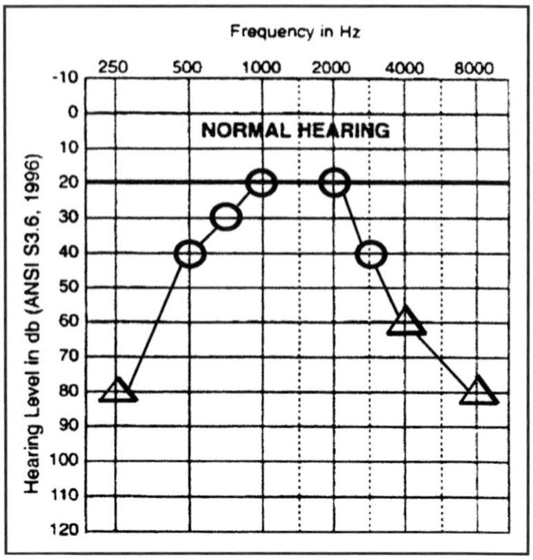

B

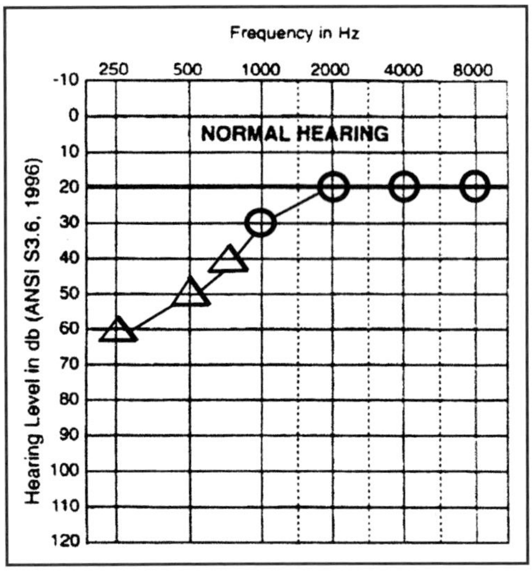

C

Fig 7–1. Examples of pure-tone threshold patterns seen in patients with Ménière's disease.

lesser magnitude. It should be noted that total hearing loss as a result of Ménière's disease is rare, and its presence should arouse suspicion of another diagnosis (eg, genetic, syphilitic, autoimmune).

Fluctuations in hearing, particularly in the low frequencies during the early stages of the disorder, are noted in 50 to 70% of patients.[4,5] Thus, in the early stages of the disorder, patients may present with a history of vertigo and symptoms of unilateral auditory dysfunction, yet the audiogram is normal. Alternatively, the audiogram may only reveal a high-frequency hearing loss. These findings result from the low-frequency hearing loss resolving after an acute episode. Although these findings may cloud the diagnosis early on in the disease process, the audiometric picture may be clarified by having the patient present for audiometric assessment during a period of acute exacerbation. With time, the low-frequency hearing loss will become persistent and the ambiguity of the early audiometric findings will be resolved.

Electrocochleography

Electrocochleography (ECOG) is a form of evoked potential audiometry that has had particular application to the evaluation of patients with Ménière's disease. As we will see from the following discussion, some of the assumptions made about the interpretation of ECOG recording must be questioned in light of current evidence and the role of ECOG in the evaluation of patients is uncertain.

Electrocochleography is the recording of electrical activity of cochlear hair cells and auditory nerve elicited by either broad spectrum sound clicks or more frequency-specific tone bursts.[6–8] The active recording electrode may be placed through the tympanic membrane onto the cochlear promontory (transtympanic recording) or on the surface of the tympanic membrane (extratympanic recording). Three different potentials are recorded by electrocochleography —the cochlear microphonic (CM), the compound action potential (AP), and the summating potential (SP).

The cochlear microphonic is an AC potential that represents the electrical activity within outer hair cells when they are subjected to a prolonged auditory stimulus. The CM generally is not recorded for clinical purposes and, in fact, stimuli are configured to avoid CM interference with SP and AP recording. The cochlear compound action potential (AP) represents the sum of the electrical activity from multiple, simultaneously firing cochlear nerve afferent fibers. It is analogous to wave I of the auditory brainstem response (ABR). The summating potential (SP) is a DC potential. During acoustic stimulation, hair cells repeatedly depolarize and repolarize in response to basilar membrane motion. Throughout these cycles of depolarization and repolarization, the magnitude of cellular depolarization is greater than the magnitude of cellular repolarization. That is, the hair cell does not return to its resting potential until the auditory stimulus ceases. The failure of the hair cell to completely repolarize creates a DC potential that represents the difference between the magnitude of the cell's normal resting potential and the potential it achieves during repolarization. The sum of these DC potentials generated in individual hair cells is what we record as the SP (Fig 7–2).

Electrocochleography and Ménière's Disease

Elevations in the SP in patients with Ménière's disease have long been described.[9] Greater accuracy was derived by measuring the ratio of the amplitude of the SP and the amplitude of the AP[10] and this has remained the measure of choice in evoked potential audiometry when evaluating patients with possible Ménière's disease.

A large number of clinical studies document elevations in the SP/AP ratio in a significant number of patients with Ménière's disease.[6,11–16] However, sufficient issues exist pertaining to the

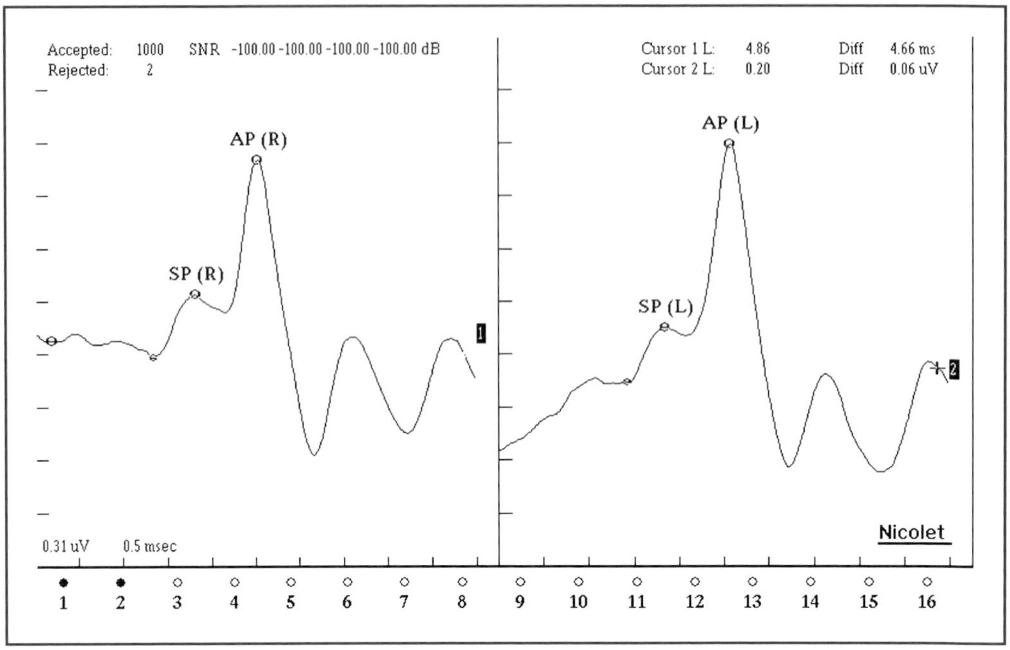

Fig 7–2. Examples of SP and AP recordings obtained using a click stimulus from the right and left ears of the same patient. (SP = Summating Potential; AP =Action Potential).

recording, interpretation, and sensitivity of this test to result in questioning its utility in routine clinical diagnostic regimens.

- *Transtympanic versus extratympanic recording.* Outside North America, placing the recording electrode through the tympanic membrane so that it rests on the promontory (transtympanic placement) is the favored recording technique. Transtympanic recording provides a very robust signal to noise ratio, thus decreasing the variability in recordings and decreasing the time required to achieve a good quality waveform. It does require a physician to place the electrode and obviously involves a degree of invasiveness. A recording electrode can also be placed in the ear canal adjacent to the tympanic membrane (extratympanic recording) or directly on the tympanic membrane. This is a less invasive technique and a physician is not required to place the electrode, but using this method results in a compromise in the quality and reproducibility of the waveforms. Perhaps more importantly, the increase in signal strength elicited by transtympanic recording is not equally distributed to the SP and the AP. That is, the SP recorded using the transtympanic technique is 4 times greater than that recorded with an extratympanic electrode, while the AP is 6 times greater when transtympanic recordings are compared to extratympanic recordings.[17] Thus, when establishing norms for the SP/AP, data derived from transtympanic studies cannot be directly compared to data derived from extratympanic recordings (see below).

- *Stimulus type.* A broadband click has been classically used to record the SP and AP. Tone bursts, which are more frequency specific than a click stimulus, have also been used based on the rationale that they can stimulate more specific areas of the cochlea, thus allowing for greater focus on areas that may be affected by the pathology. There is some evidence that recording responses to tonebursts may improve diagnostic sensitivity.[18] A transtympanic electrode is generally required to reliably record responses to toneburst stimuli. This is due, in part, to a loss of some synchronicity of neural firing due to the longer duration of the toneburst stimulus.
- *Stimulus and recording parameters.* It must be emphasized that changes in the stimulus and recording parameters can result in significant differences in waveform morphology and temporal patterns. Perusal of the literature reveals significant variation in these parameters when comparing various studies. Thus, care must be taken when comparing data derived from different studies.
- *Interinterpreter variability in defining the SP.* The examples of electrocochleography waveforms provided above reveal a very obvious SP. However, this is not always the case. The SP can prove difficult to identify, resulting in potential errors in calculating the SP/AP. In fact, there can be significant interinterpreter differences in SP/AP ratios calculated from the same tracing.[19] This has considerable implications pertaining to the reliability of the test if it is to be used routinely in a clinical setting.
- *What constitutes an abnormal SP/AP?* Perhaps the greatest issue pertaining to the use of electrocochleography as a diagnostic tool is what constitutes an abnormal SP/AP. In a meta-analysis, Wuyts and colleagues determined that SP/AP of 0.35 derived using **transtympanic** recordings would reasonably discriminate between normal patients and those with Ménière's disease.[8] **Extratympanic** recordings reveal a broader deviation about the mean and, as such, an accurate determination of what constitutes an abnormal SP/AP was more difficult to derive. The authors concluded that an SP/AP of 0.42 recorded with an extratympanic electrode reasonably separated normal patients from patients with Ménière's disease.
- *Is the test valid?* If electrocochleography is to be a meaningful diagnostic test, then there must be a clear delineation between normal and abnormal results. The test must be validated by traditional epidemiological

measures of *sensitivity* and *specificity*. Furthermore, if the test is to be valuable, it must not just be abnormal in cases of obvious, established Ménière's disease. In this case, it would only be confirming the obvious. Ideally, it should be able to confirm a diagnosis in an ambiguous case, such as in an early case where the patient may present with some but not all the symptoms (eg, fluctuating hearing loss with no vertigo or recurrent vertigo with no hearing loss).

Studies done to validate electrocochleography have determined its sensitivity to be a modest 55 to 65%.[9,15,20–24] The sensitivity may be augmented by also calculating the SP/AP in response to toneburst stimuli.[23] It must be emphasized that these statistics were derived in patients carrying a diagnosis of "definite" Ménière's disease. In cases of possible Ménière's disease, it is even less predictive, with a sensitivity as low as 20% in cases of early Ménière's disease.

The diagnosis of Ménière's disease is made based on clinical criteria. If the patient definitely meets the diagnostic criteria of Ménière's disease, then why do we require a test to confirm what is already clear? This question must be applied particularly in the case of electrocochleography, which demonstrates a mediocre sensitivity. There certainly are cases where the diagnosis of Ménière's disease is in doubt, and being able to confirm the diagnosis would be helpful both for determining the patient's prognosis and for instituting an appropriate treatment regimen. However, the sensitivity offered by electrocochleography, even when augmented by toneburst stimuli, does not allow this test to confirm an ambiguous diagnosis.

- *Can electrocochleography diagnose endolymphatic hydrops?* As described above, there is no question that elevations in the SP/AP do occur in patients with Ménière's disease. However, it must be emphasized that these studies draw an association between these findings in electrocochleography and the clinical entity of Ménière's disease. It is quite remarkable that it has become accepted in much of the audiologic and clinical otolaryngologic literature that alterations in the SP/AP ratio provide scientific evidence for the presence of hydrops within the cochlea. Such conclusions are simply unfounded. Basic scientific studies on animals with induced endolymphatic hydrops provide the only manner in which electrocochleographic recordings can be made and then immediately correlated with morphological abnormalities within the cochlea. These animals develop profound hydrops, which can be documented on histological analysis. A number of well-controlled studies from laboratories with extensive expertise in the hydrops model have now been performed, which have analyzed changes in cochlear potentials in animals with well-established hydrops.[25,26] These studies have been consistent in failing to report any significant alterations in the SP or the SP/AP ratio in animals with hydrops. Thus, alterations in the SP or the SP/AP ratio may be correlated with the clinical entity of Ménière's disease, but they are note related to the presence or degree of hydrops.

Conclusions Regarding Electrocochleography and Ménière's Disease

The SP/AP ratio can be elevated in a significant number of patients with Ménière's disease. However, the sensitivity of the test is only 55 to 65% in cases of definite Ménière's disease, and it is worse in early cases of the disorder. Thus, at present, it is difficult to recommend the test for use in the routine clinical evaluation of patients with possible Ménière's disease. Furthermore, although abnormalities in the SP/AP ratio are seen in patients with Ménière's disease, these abnormalities are not correlated with the presence of endolymphatic hydrops as demonstrated by data obtained in animal models.

References

1. Barber HO. Ménière's disease: symptomatology. In: Oosterveld WJ, ed. *Ménière's Disease: A Comprehensive Appraisal.* New York, NY: John Wiley & Sons; 1983:25–34.
2. Stahle J, Friberg U, Svedberg A. Long-term progression of Ménière's disease. *Acta Otolaryngol Suppl.* 1991;485:78–83.
3. Katsarkis A. Hearing loss and vestibular dysfunction in Ménière's disease. *Acta Otolaryngol (Stockh).* 1996;116:185–188.
4. Green JD Jr, Blum DJ, Harner SG. Longitudinal followup of patients with Ménière's disease. *Otolaryngol Head Neck Surg.* 1991;104(6):783–788.
5. Haye R, Quist-Hanssen S. The natural course of Ménière's disease. *Acta Otolaryngol.* 1976;82(3–4):289–293.
6. Ferraro JA, Durrant JD. Electrocochleography in the evaluation of patients with Ménière's disease/endolymphatic hydrops. *J Am Acad Audiol.* 2006;17(1): 45–68.
7. Wuyts FL, Van de Heyning PH, Van Spaendonck MP, Molenberghs G. A review of electrocochleography: instrumentation settings and meta-analysis of criteria for diagnosis of endolymphatic hydrops. *Acta Otolaryngol Suppl.* 1997;526:14–20.
8. Wuyts FL, Van de Heyning PH, Van Spaendonck M, et al. Rate influences on tone burst summating potential amplitude in electrocochleography: clinical(a) and experimental(b) data. *Hear Res.* 2001;152(1–2):1–9.
9. Gibson WP, Moffat DA, Ramsden RT. Clinical electrocochleography in the diagnosis and management of Ménière's disorder. *Audiology.* 1977;16(5):389–401.
10. Eggermont JJ. Summating potentials in electrocochleography: relation to hearing disorders. In: Ruben RJ, Eiberling C, Salomon G, eds. *Electrocochleography.* Baltimore, MD: University Park Press; 1976:67–88.
11. Dauman R, Cazals Y, Aran JM. Frequency selectivity: reliability of electrocochleographic measures with iso-intensity masking. *Acta Otolaryngol.* 1988;105(1–2): 50–55.

12. Goin DW, Staller SJ, Asher DL, Mischke RE. Summating potential in Ménière's disease. *Laryngoscope.* 1982;92(12):1383–1389.
13. Morrison AW, Moffat DA, O'Connor AF. Clinical usefulness of electrocochleography in Ménière's disease: an analysis of dehydrating agents. *Otolaryngol Clin North Am.* 1980;13(4):703–721.
14. Ruth RA, Lambert PR, Ferraro JA. Electrocochleography: methods and clinical applications. *Am J Otol.* 1988;9(suppl): 1–11.
15. Coats AC. The summating potential and Ménière's disease. I. Summating potential amplitude in Ménière and non-Ménière ears. *Arch Otolaryngol.* 1981; 107(4):199–208.
16. Ohashi T, Takeyama I. Clinical significance of SP/AP ratio in inner ear diseases. *ORL J Otorhinolaryngol Relat Spec.* 1989;51(4):235–245.
17. Ferraro JA, Thedinger BS, Mediavilla SJ, Blackwell WL. Human summating potential to tone bursts: observations on tympanic membrane versus promontory recordings in the same patients. *J Am Acad Audiol.* 1994;5(1):24–29.
18. Conlon BJ, Gibson WP. Electrocochleography in the diagnosis of Ménière's disease. *Acta Otolaryngol.* 2000;120(4): 480–483.
19. Roland PS, Roth L. Interinterpreter variability in determining the SP/AP ratio in clinical electrocochleography. *Laryngoscope.* 1997;107(10):1357–1361.
20. Ferraro JA, Tibbils RP. SP/AP area ratio in the diagnosis of Ménière's disease. *Am J Audiol.* 1999;8(1):21–28.
21. Margolis RH, Rieks D, Fournier EM, Levine SE. Tympanic electrocochleography for diagnosis of Ménière's disease. *Arch Otolaryngol Head Neck Surg.* 1995;121(1):44–55.
22. Kim HH, Wiet RJ, Battista RA. Trends in the diagnosis and the management of Ménière's disease: results of a survey. *Otolaryngol Head Neck Surg.* 2005;132(5): 722–726.
23. Sass K. Sensitivity and specificity of transtympanic electrocochleography in Ménière's disease. *Acta Otolaryngol.* 1998;118(2):150–156.
24. Pou AM, Hirsch BE, Durrant JD, Gold SR, Kamerer DB. The efficacy of tympanic electrocochleography in the diagnosis of endolymphatic hydrops. *Am J Otol.* 1996;17(4):607–611.
25. Salt AN, DeMott J. Time course of endolymph volume increase in experimental hydrops measured in vivo with an ionic volume marker. *Hear Res.* 1994; 74(1–2):165–172.
26. Horner KC. Auditory and vestibular function in experimental hydrops. *Otolaryngol Head Neck Surg.* 1995;112(1): 84–89.

8

Vestibular and Balance Function Testing

Neil T. Shepard

Introduction

Vestibular function and balance testing is a necessary component of the investigation of a patient with known or suspected Ménière's syndrome. The rationale for this statement comes not from specific test findings that are unique to Ménière's, as there are no currently known unique findings or combinations for Ménière's. The purpose for the testing grows out of the need to: (1) determine the status of the peripheral vestibular system thought to be involved; (2) determine the status of the contralateral system; (3) investigate general balance ability between the events of vertigo; (4) assist in ruling out central vestibular system causes for the dizziness; and (5) assist in the monitoring of the effectiveness of certain treatments. The testing findings, when interpreted in the context of hearing loss and the presenting symptoms, develop a profile that can be used to assist in the determination of the diagnosis of Ménière's. This chapter concentrates on what tools for vestibular and balance function assessment are available and how their interpretation can be of assistance in both the diagnosis and management of the Ménière's patient. Prior to that discussion further consideration of the five purposes listed above is needed.

Although it is not included in the formal definition of Ménière's syndrome from the American Academy of Otolaryngology-Head and Neck Surgery,[1] an expected part of the profile of a patient with Ménière's would be the development, possible fluctuation of and progression of a peripheral vestibular hypofunction on the side involved. The vestibular function studies of caloric irrigations, rotational chair, and the use of vestibular evoked myogenic potential (VEMP) provide for this monitoring. Even though there is not a unique pattern for Ménière's in these studies, there are patterns that apparently have an increased likelihood of being associated with Ménière's, such a hypofunction with an irritative status and changes in the most sensitive frequency response to VEMP testing with tone bursts (discussed in detail below). The recognition of these situations and the progressive nature of a peripheral hypofunction can assist in differentiating Ménière's from other disorders and, importantly, from migraine headaches, which can present with the same symptoms including a mild hypofunction.[2,3]

In considering treatment options, especially aggressive pathways that will deliberately cause damage to the affected side, knowledge of the contralateral vestibular system is of importance. Making sure it is functioning adequately and that there are no signs of possible development of a Ménière's process on the contralateral side or indications of damage from past insults influence the management option decisions.

When investigating the general status of functional balance, indications of symptoms of dizziness proved by head movement become important to characterize the need for vestibular and balance therapy as a management tool between the spontaneous events of dizziness. Residual symptoms between the Ménière's attacks can be managed with vestibular and balance therapy, especially if risks for falls is involved. It needs to be clearly understood that the use of such a therapy program will have no impact on the spontaneous events of Ménière's attacks but only on the residual symptoms. For details of the use of vestibular and balance therapy, see Chapter 12 in this text.

Another purpose in the use of vestibular function testing is the screening for possible central vestibular system involvement via pursuit tracking, saccade testing and gaze stability.[4] The typical profile for a Ménière's patient would not include any indications of central vestibular system involvement. It has been reported that in severe cases of Ménière's syndrome indications of cerebellar involvement can be seen through abnormal pursuit tracking.[5] However, in this work the patients were not screened for migraine. It is well documented that not only peripheral but also indications of central vestibular system involvement are seen via pursuit tracking and gaze stability testing in active migraine patients.[6,7] The issue of migraine is especially important as the estimated life time prevalence of migraine headache disorder in well-documented Ménière's patients exceeds 50%.[8]

The fifth and final purpose for the use of vestibular function testing in Ménière's patients is that of monitoring of the effects of certain treatment options. In management activities that involve the use of titration of gentamicin, monitoring the physiologic impact of the drug on the affected side can be useful in determining when to stop the drug in addition to patient symptoms. If symptoms seem to be continuing following the use of a vestibular nerve section, labyrinthectomy, or with gentamicin, investigation of the physiologic status of the peripheral system involved can be of significant assistance in planning the next course of action. The investigation tools now available allow for not only monitoring horizontal semicircular canal via caloric and rotational chair protocol, but also quantifying the status of the saccule and utricle.[9]

Specific Test Selection and Interpretation

Routine Tests of Vestibular Function

To accomplish the purposes listed above, there are a variety of routine and some nonroutine studies that maybe selected for use. As an initial investigation, not all studies available may be needed (ie, rotational chair may not add any information to the patient that has a hypofunction by caloric irrigation testing and spontaneous and positional nystagmus that is beating away from the hypofunction). However, if a patient is going to be offered a treatment activity that involves more than the conservative low salt diet and diuretic, use of rotational chair would be useful in establishing a baseline to follow the progress of the treatment over time. It would be especially useful in the transtympanic gentamicin treatment option. In the patient when no indications of spontaneous or positional nystagmus is seen and caloric testing is normal, the use of rotational chair to expand the investigation of the peripheral system for indications of labyrinthine involvement can be very helpful. The use of a staged protocol, as implied in this discussion, allows for what is needed on the patient for initial investigation or setting baseline for monitoring treatment but uses only the tests needed to accomplish that purpose without overtesting the patient. A full discussion of the use of a staged protocol can be found elsewhere and is not repeated here.[10,11]

The routine studies that should be used on any patient to assist in the initial investigation of a suspected Ménière's patient would involve a typical electronystagmography (ENG)/videonystagmography (VNG) protocol. A general discussion of the administration of and general interpretation of the ENG/VNG and other less routine tests discussed below is provided elsewhere in detail.[12] Included in the ENG/VNG protocol should be the ocular motor evaluations of pursuit tracking, random individual eye saccade testing, and gaze stability, all to characterize the status of the central vestibular system to rule out its involvement. Dix-Hallpike testing is used for review of presence of benign paroxysmal positional vertigo (BPPV), which is not uncommon in individuals with other peripheral disorders independent of the etiology. Spontaneous and positional nystagmus, although not localizing in general, can be of use in a Ménière's patient if it is direction fixed as it can suggest an irritative status to the suspected peripheral system involved. This can be especially important if the caloric testing shows a hypofunction on the suspected side. Then the combination of nystagmus beating toward the hypofunctional side indicates a paretic lesion with an irritative status, a condition seen in Ménière's patients most often in the early onset of the disorder.[3] A case example illustrates this situation.

Case 1

This 34-year-old female reported with documented fluctuations in hearing on the left with indications of slow progression of mild to moderate hearing loss of sensorineural nature on the left, especially in the frequency range below 2 kHz. Hearing on the right was within normal limits and she had no auditory complaints on the right. The hearing difficulties had been ongoing for about 1.5 years. Over the last 12 months, she had begun to experience spontaneous events of true vertigo lasting from 15 minutes to 4 hours with nausea and vomiting accompanied with imbalance that would extend into the next day. She would then return to her normal baseline other than her hearing loss. She reported increases in tinnitus and aural fullness on the left with the events of vertigo. The spontaneous events had been as frequent as one per week but at time of initial investigation were about 2 per month. Her VNG showed normal ocular motor testing with no gaze nystagmus with fixation present. When fixation was removed, she had a spontaneous left beating nystagmus ranging from 3 to 5 degrees/sec. This was seen throughout the study in all positions. Bithermal alternating caloric open water irrigations showed a 73% left reduced vestibular response with a 36% left directional preponderance (corrected for spontaneous). Absolute responses from the left to warm and ice water were 3 to 7 degrees per sec all left beating. On the right, the responses were 11 to 40 degrees per sec for warm and ice water irrigations. These studies indicate a left hypofunction with an irritative status. Because nystagmus always beats toward the more active neural side, the left-beating spontaneous nystagmus and the left directional preponderance indicate that the left side had the greater intrinsic neural activity. The caloric test then is giving information about the peripheral vestibular system's ability to respond to an extrinsic stimulus (the water irrigation) and that result indicates that the left vestibular periphery responds significantly less than the right. It is unusual to see an irritative status, especially in the context of that same periphery having a hypofunction response, but this is a condition that can be seen in Ménière's patients. The work by Maire and van Miller[3] as well as others[13,14] shows that, during and between the spontaneous events, the affected side will change from an irritative to paretic status.

In a situation as illustrated in case 1, the combined use of the direction of the spontaneous nystagmus together with the caloric results were of use in defining a situation that would be most consistent with Ménière's. Outside the opportunity to see an irritative status with normal caloric results (spontaneous and positional nystagmus beating toward the suspected involved side with hearing loss), and the situation illustrated in case 1, no other patterns on the routine testing within an ENG/VNG apparently are most consistent with Ménière's. The more common pattern of results from an ENG/VNG also is one seen in a variety of peripherally involved processes where positional nystagmus is present with normal ocular motor testing and a hypofunction by caloric testing may or may not be present. If present, the nystagmus, if direction fixed, would beat away from the hypofunction—a classic paretic lesion pattern. In that case, the lack of central findings and the presence of peripheral involvement on the suspected side (the side with the documented hearing loss of a progressive nature) would be consistent with possible Ménière's but not unique to Ménière's. In a situation of this type, the presence of the progressive hearing loss with documented fluctuations is critically necessary to connect the indications of peripheral vestibular system involvement and the presenting symptoms of spontaneous events of vertigo to a possible diagnosis of Ménière's. Without the hearing loss, the likelihood that the peripheral vestibular involvement is that of Ménière's syndrome is reduced. A second case example is illustrative of this situation.

Case 2

This 62-year-old female reported a 6-year history of right side aural fullness, tinnitus, and fluctuant hearing loss of mild degree. These symptoms were in the context of spontaneous events of vertigo that would last from 1 to 6 hours occurring once every 2 to 3 months but over the last 6 months had occurred once per month. The events would occur without headache but about 50% did occur with photophobia. Her past medical history was positive for migraine headaches that had improved substantially with menopause and were occurring no more frequently than one per month and easily handled with over-the-counter pain medication for migraine. She did report scintillating scatomas which fit the criteria for ocular migraines and would occur once every 3 to 4 months. Her hearing tests over the last 6 years had always showed normal hearing even when performed shortly after a vertigo event and during times when she felt hearing was diminished. ENG was well within normal limits for ocular motor testing and showed no indications of spontaneous or positional nystagmus with negative Dix-Hallpike testing. In her case, rotational chair testing (discussed below) also was negative. Her caloric testing did show a 28% right reduced vestibular response with normal directional preponderance. Based on the above findings and her history, her working diagnosis was Ménière's syndrome on the right. She was seen for a second opinion as conservative treatments had been of no assistance and recommendations for more aggressive treatments had been suggested. On further, testing hearing continued to be within normal limits, now 6 years from the start of the spells of vertigo. Her repeat VNG showed a 30% right reduced vestibular response with all other subtests within the VNG normal. Secondary to the lack of any evidence of hearing loss over the 6-year interval, the diagnosis of Ménière's syndrome on the right was substantially in doubt. Given the consistency with which she would experience photophobia with her vertigo events and her past diagnosis of migraine headaches, the possibility of her dizziness being migraine related was entertained. She subsequently was treated for migraine headaches with dietary changes and prophylactic medication and her events of vertigo along with the auditory complaints resolved.

In case 2, the right hypofunction together with the symptom complaints would have been appropriate to support a possible Ménière's with the exception that, over time, no change in hearing was appreciated. The significant relationship between migraine and Ménière's[8] and the well-documented changes that can occur in vestibular function with migraine, including mild hypofunction[6] caused the impression of Ménière's in this case. This case presents a prime example of how the vestibular function tests require interpretation in the context of not only the presenting symptoms but in the case of Ménière's the hearing test results over time. A full discussion of this differentiation between Ménière's and migraine and the confusion that can exist as both can occur together is provided in other literature[2] and is outside the scope of this chapter.

As a lead in to the use of other tests that we will refer to as nonroutine, the situation of having fully normal findings on an ENG/VNG in the presence of a well focused symptom presentation appropriate for Ménière's together with documented fluctuations and progressive loss of hearing is not inconsistent with Ménière's syndrome. Early in the onset of the disorder and contingent on the severity and frequency of the spells of vertigo, a patient may well go a year or longer with insufficient permanent damage to the peripheral vestibular system that can be recognized with clinically significant nystagmus or abnormal caloric findings.[3] It is a situation of this nature that fosters the use for other studies of vestibular function that would be considered supplemental to the ENG/VNG series of subtests. Additionally, three specific electrophysiologic studies have been developed specifically for the attempt to find results that would be unique to Ménière's syndrome. Two of theses would be electrocochleography (ECoG) and cochlear hydrops auditory measurement procedure (CHAMP), which deal directly with the changes in the cochlea as a result of Ménière's. These are beyond the scope of this chapter and the interested reader is referred to Chapter 7 on audiologic function. The third electrophysiologic technique is use of vestibular evoked myogenic potentials (VEMP) for investigation of the saccule. Given that Ménière's is referred to as a cochleosaccular disorder and that the endolymphatic hydrops can be seen in both the cochlea and saccule (see Chapters 3 and 4) VEMP testing is considered in detail below.

Nonroutine Tests of Vestibular System Function

The following tests are referred to as nonroutine not because they are obscure but secondary to lack of availability in facilities that would have ready access to ENG/VNG.

Rotational Chair Protocols

The use of rotational chair step tests or sinusoidal protocols are both means to expand the investigation of the peripheral vestibular system.[15] There is no specific pattern of findings that are suggestive of Ménière's, but abnormalities suggestive of peripheral vestibular system involvement can be useful in making a case for labyrinthine involvement in the context of an appropriate history, especially if the ENG/VNG testing is normal. Another use of the rotational chair is during treatment, especially with transtympanic gentamicin injections, to monitor status of the peripheral system via changes in phase angle (time constant) and symmetry values.[16] Although not unique to Ménière's, the issue of bilateral vestibular system involvement and its extent requires the use of total body rotation for defining this situation.[8] Last, the quantitative assessment of the utricle is a study requiring a controlled force to be placed on the utricular organ right versus left. This requires the use of a specially designed rotational chair with the capability of moving the position of the chair so the axis of rotation can be placed through either the right or left utricular system.[9,17] As with the other functions of rotational chair, the findings are not known to be unique to Ménière's but again add a new dimension of peripheral system investigation. This specific investigation of the utricular system may prove very useful in the patient thought to be suffering from crisis of Tumarkin events.[18,19]

Postural Control Assessment

The principle purpose of this investigative avenue with sensory organization testing [20] is the functional assessment of the maintenance of static and dynamic quiet stance. This allows for a characterization of the functional impact Ménière's or other peripheral system lesions have on a patient's balance. To that end, the test can be of use in recommending vestibular and balance rehabilitation therapy for the residual symptoms between the vertiginous events. The various other protocols, motor control testing, postural evoked responses and platform pressure testing,[20] are useful in a variety of central and other labyrinthine lesions find little utility in Ménière's syndrome.

Vestibular Evoked Myogenic Potential Ttesting (VEMP)

A full generic discussion of VEMP testing is beyond the scope of this chapter and the interested reader is referred to work by Atkin and Murnane, 2008[21] for a thorough summary. Because VEMP is a specific investigation of the saccule and the saccule appears as a major component of effect of Ménière's, considerable effort has been put into looking for unique markers of the VEMP test in a Ménière's population.[22–24] Another application of VEMPs to Ménière's is with the use of VEMP thresholds to tone bursts of 250, 500, 750 Hz and 1 kHz and a click to supplement the information of hearing studies and caloric irrigations for early detection of the involved side.[25] This work did show an improvement of early detection of the correct Ménière's side with the addition of the threshold information to that obtained from the caloric irrigation testing and the information from hearing testing. An expanded use of the VEMP thresholds at 250, 500, 750 Hz and 1 kHz producing a VEMP threshold response curve ("tuning curve") are the shape changes in the curves most sensitive frequency in an active Ménière's ear.[26] When the threshold in dB SPL peak of the tone burst is plotted as a function of frequency the most sensitive frequency is generally 500 Hz.[26,27] In Ménière's patients, the most sensitive frequency has been shown to shift upward with an elevation in threshold level.[26]

A further finding has been that in about 50% of those with unilateral Ménière's changes in the threshold response curve of a similar nature were noted in the asymptomatic ear, raising the possibility of early detection of developing Ménière's in those who may be bilateral for the disorder.[26] In further work, the suggestion of being able to detect the development in the contralateral ear in about 30% of the patient's studied was further supported.[28] It also has been shown that the magnitude of the changes in the shape and elevation of thresholds is directly proportional to the severity of the disorder as indicated by the presence of Tumarkin crisis events as an indicator of end stage of Ménière's syndrome.[29] Although these changes noted in the VEMP threshold response curve are exciting as a potential real-time marker for Ménière's, it must be considered a work in progress at this time. The one element that is missing is completion of a study showing that the changes noted thus far in Ménière's patients are unique to that group and not seen in other peripheral vestibular disorders.

Potential Impact of Proximity of a Ménière's Attack to the Vestibular Testing

A case example is used to illustrate the potential influence of the effect of a recent Ménière's attack on the vestibular test results.

Case 3

This 48-year-old female had a longstanding history of fluctuant hearing on the left with documented progressive loss of a sensorineural nature. She had been having spontaneous spells of vertigo that would last from 1 to 4 hours and occurred approximately once every 4 to 6 months over a several year interval. Hearing on the right was normal and past vestibular function studies had indicated a mild left hypofunction. In the 8 months prior to being seen, her vertigo events had increase to a frequency of 1 to 3 times per month. She subsequently was seen for review of more aggressive options for management. Two days prior to her vestibular testing, she had a major Ménière's attack with 4 hours of vertigo, nausea, vomiting, and significant transient loss of hearing on the left. The event started very suddenly with an apparent Tumarkin crisis causing a sudden fall with injury and then the vertigo and other symptoms began. The testing revealed a persistent left-beating nystagmus of a spontaneous nature throughout the VNG with fixation removed. No nystagmus was noted with fixation present and her pursuit and saccade testing was normal. Her caloric testing showed all four water caloric irrigations to result in absolute nystagmus slow component velocities between 6 to 10° per sec. This is an indication of possible bilateral vestibular involvement. Outside ENG, 12 months prior, had shown values on the right side in the range of 15 to 25° per sec.

Her rotational chair testing using the sinusoidal protocol indicated an increased phase lead of a modest magnitude (60°) at 0.01 Hz with normal gain and a right greater than left slow component asymmetry (suggestive of an irritative status) at multiple frequencies from 0.01 to 0.16 Hz. She reported no auditory symptoms on the right and her VEMP threshold response curve was normal for the right side with no responses on the left at any tone burst frequency. The suspicion was that, because she had the last event of significance ending within 48 hours of the testing, the central compensation system was within a static compensation phase [30] that would cause the system to appear as a bilateral mild low-frequency hypofunction. The other clue was that if this was a true bilateral hypofunction, even mild low frequency, from pathologic insult, we would have expected the phase lead on rotational chair to be in the a range from 68° or greater. Therefore, a treatment of transtympanic steroid was applied to her left ear. She then returned for follow up in 6 weeks and reported that the injection had seem to quiet the events such that she went 3 weeks with no vertigo event; however, within the last 3 weeks, she had 5 events. The last one was 10 days prior to her return visit. At the return visit, caloric testing was repeated, now showing a significant left hypofunction with responses in the 5 to 7° per sec range on the left and 20 to 26° per sec on the right. Rotational chair testing continued to show increased phase lead at 0.01 Hz of 62° with normal gain and a left greater than right asymmetry at all frequencies tested (consistent with a left hypofunction). She subsequently was treated with gentamicin and, over a 2-month interval, her vertiginous events stopped and she has now been vertigo-free for over 12 months.

In case 3, the concern that arose was the possibility of onset of bilateral involvement given the finding from the caloric testing. However, the chair results were not consistent with bilateral peripheral pathology in that the phase lead was not of a significant enough magnitude to be convincing of true bilateral involvement. In a situation of this nature, had there been other indications of involvement in the previously uninvolved ear, then the bilateral indications would have been taken with a greater weighting as that could have influenced the future treatment options. However, given the lack of any other indicators that the contralateral ear was starting into participation in Ménière's and the fact that the phase lead on rotational chair was too modest for bilateral involvement, it strongly suggested that this was a false bilateral indication. At the return visit and at subsequent visits, it was definitely supported that the result was a false bilateral indication via the normal caloric response that was seen in the uninvolved ear. The purpose of presenting case 3 is to draw attention to the fact that, when testing a Ménière's patient, the results need to be interpreted in the context of when the most recent Ménière's attack occurred. It will vary; however, if an event of significance has occurred within the last 48 hours and possibly within the last 72, the residual effects may influence the test results seen. The most likely effect would be that of abnormal postural control results, but as in the case above, the indications for a false bilateral weakness can be seen. This is not to suggest that testing shortly following an event is inappropriate but rather that careful interpretation, taking the timing and other symptom information into account, is critical in the final interpretation of the test findings. Nor does case 3 suggest that rotational chair testing is a requirement for each Ménière's patient being seen. If rotational chair is routinely available, then it should be incorporated in the definition that is used for bilateral hypofunction for the magnitude of the phase angle, even if the gain values are normal. If the chair testing is not available, then caution should be exercised in suggesting bilateral involvement based on caloric alone when other features are not consistent. If there is a history of a recent spell and the test results are suggesting bilateral involvement without other indicators, repeating of the caloric irrigations in another 2 to 3 days could be very telling.

There are situations where testing shortly after a vertigo event may be beneficial as you are more likely to see nystagmus direction for spontaneous or positional testing have the beat toward the known involved side indicative of an irritative style lesion.[3]

Case 4

A 37-year-old male reported the onset of vertigo lasting 1 to 2 days over the last 1.5 years and a progressive change in his hearing on the right with tinnitus and occasional aural fullness. Vestibular and balance testing was negative for any indications of central vestibular system involvement and showed no spontaneous or positional nystagmus on the day of testing but did demonstrate a 32% right reduced vestibular response. Rotational chair showed normal gains with an increase phase lead at 0.01 and 0.04 Hz with a mild right greater than left slow component asymmetry at 0.01 and 0.04 Hz. VEMP threshold response curves were normal bilaterally and an outside electrocochleography study was borderline for the right and clearly negative for the left. Postural control was normal. The patient had a working diagnosis of Ménière's on the right with no effect of conservative treatments of low sodium diet with diuretic and no effect of steroid injection times 2 in the right. The vertigo events were 1 to 3 per month and the patient had been recommended to have gentamicin injections for control of the symptoms and had presented for a second opinion. Under further detailed questioning about his spells of vertigo, it was revealed that on the 1- to 2-day intervals when the symptoms were present the occurred only with head movements even though the initial description from the patient was simply a 1- to 2-day interval with vertigo nausea, and vomiting. When questioned closely it was clear that the vertigo would last only 1 to 2 minutes at most provoked by head movements during these 1- to 2-day intervals of symptoms. He would experience general nausea continuously during the symptomatic interval with significant photophobia but denied associated headaches. He had a long-standing history of migraine headaches over the last 10 years with only modest control with headache multiple times per month that met the international headache society criteria for migraine.

It also was reported that he denied any fluctuations in hearing on either side and that the sensorineural loss of hearing (generally flat configuration) on the right was a very slow progressive loss that had begun some 10 years before with documented hearing tests dating to that time. He denied any change in auditory symptoms with his intervals of head movement provoked vertigo. His family history revealed his father and father's brother both with hearing loss in the right ear documented by hearing tests. The patient had a normal contrasted MRI with an internal auditory canal protocol. Given that his symptoms were that of head movement provoked vertigo lasting seconds to minutes that would occur in spontaneous intervals of hours to 2 days, accompanied with photophobia instead of spontaneous spells of vertigo lasting hours, the alternative diagnosis to Ménière's of migraine-related dizziness with hereditary hearing loss was entertained. It was speculated that the abnormal findings on the vestibular testing was probably migraine in origin[6] and that he met the definition of migraine related dizziness as proposed by Neuhauser et al, 2001.[31] As a result, he was aggressively treated with dietary restrictions and a prophylactic medication for migraine and at his 6-month return visit he had remained without vertigo or headache symptoms since a month after stating the migraine treatment. At that point, his diagnosis was formally changed to migraine-related dizziness with familial unilateral sensorineural hearing loss.

Case 4 is a good example of the difficulty that can arise when the test findings, including auditory and vestibular, used to support a history that was not fully consistent with Ménière's for the diagnosis of Ménière's syndrome. This brings us back to the principal thrust of this chapter in that vestibular and balance testing, although helpful in the Ménière's patient, must be matched with the other Ménière's syndrome features to support that diagnosis.

Summary

This chapter summarized in detail the utilization of vestibular and balance laboratory tests in relationship to Ménière's syndrome. The nonspecific nature of the test findings to Ménière's and as a result the critical necessity to interpret the test findings in the context of the patient's presenting symptoms were discussed. Finally, the influence of the temporal proximity of a Ménière's spell on the test findings was presented in an illustrative case. The important take-home message relates to this issue of an integrated interpretation of the test findings, presenting history, and hearing loss to make the diagnosis or rule out Ménière's syndrome. Two of the cases presented demonstrated situations of a patient with Ménière's with some other complicating issue, whereas case 2 and the final case illustrate cases in which Ménière's was the incorrect diagnosis. Even though various test findings could have been consistent with Ménière's, the integrated presentation was not consistent with what would have been expected for a patient with Ménière's.

References

1. American Academy of Otolaryngology, Committee on Hearing and Equilibrium. Guidelines for the diagnosis and evaluation of therapy in Ménière's disease. *Otolaryngol Head Neck Surg.* 1995; 113:181–185.
2. Shepard NT. Differentiation of Ménière's disease and migraine associated dizziness: a review. *J Am Acad Audiol.* 2006; 17:69–80.
3. Maire R, van Melle G. Vestibulo-ocular reflex characteristics in patients with unilateral Ménière's disease. *Otol Neurotol.* 2008;29:693–698.
4. Shepard NT, Schubert M. Interpretation and usefulness of ocular motility testing. In: Jacobson GP, Shepard NT, eds. *Balance Function Assessment and Management.* San Diego, CA: Plural Publishing Inc; 2008:147–170.
5. Elina I, Heikki A, Ilmari P. Ocular motor findings mimicking a cerebellar disorder and postural control in severe Ménière's disease. *Auris Nasus Larynx.* 2008;36(1):36–41.
6. Furman JM, Marcus DA, Balaban CD. Migrainous vertigo: development of a pathogenetic model and structured diagnositic interview. *Curr Opin Neurol.* 2003;16:5–13.
7. Furman JM, Sparto PT, Soso M, Marcus D. Vestibular function in migraine-related dizziness: a pilot study. *J Vestib Res.* 2005;15:327–332.

8. Radtke A, Lempert T, Gresty MA, Brookes GB, Bronstein AM, Neuhauser H. Migraine and Ménière's disease: is there a link? *Neurology.* 2002;59:1700–1704.
9. Helling K, Schonfeld U, Clarke AH. Treatment of Ménière's disease by low-dose intratympanic gentamicin application: effect on otolith function. *Laryngoscope.* 2007;117:2244–2250.
10. Shepard NT. *Management of the Patient with Chronic Complaints of Dizziness: An Overview of Laboratory Studies.* Clackamas, OR: NeuroCom Publication; 2007.
11. Shepard NT, Telian SA. *Practical Management of the Balance Disorder Patient.* San Diego, CA: Singular Publishing Group; 1996.
12. Jacobson GP, Shepard, NT, eds. *Balance Function Assessment and Management.* San Diego, CA: Plural Publishing Inc; 2008.
13. Bance M, Mai M, Tomlinson D, Rutka J. The changing direction of nystagmus in acute Ménière's disease: pathophysiological implications. *Laryngoscope.* 1991; 101:197–201.
14. McClure JA, Copp JC, Lycett P. Recovery nystagmus in Ménière's disease. *Laryngoscope.* 1981;91:1727–1737.
15. Brey B, McPherson J, Lynch RM. Technique, interpretation and usefulness of whole body rotational testing. In: Jacobson GP, Shepard NT, eds. *Balance Function Assessment and Management.* San Diego, CA: Plural Publishing Inc; 2008:281–318.
16. Ozluoglu LN, Akkuzu G, Ozgirgin N, Tarhan E. Reliability of the vestibular evoked myogenic potential test in assessing intratympanic gentamicin therapy in Ménière's disease. *Acta Oto-Laryngol.* 2008;128(4):422–426.
17. Janky K, Shepard NT. Unilateral centrifugation: utricular assessment and protocol comparison. *Otol Neurotol.* 2010: in press.
18. Tumarkin A. The otolithic catastrophe. A new syndrome. *BMJ.* 1936;1:75–177.
19. Baloh RW, Jacobson K, Winder T. Drop attacks with Ménière's syndrome. *Ann Neurol.* 1990;28:384–387.
20. Shepard, NT. Interpretation and usefulness of computerized dynamic posturography. In: Jacobson GP, Shepard NT, eds. *Balance Function Assessment and Management.* San Diego, CA: Plural Publishing Inc; 2008: 359–378.
21. Atkin F, Murnane OD. Vestibular evoked myogenic potentials. In: Jacobson GP, Shepard NT, eds. *Balance Function Assessment and Management.* San Diego, CA: Plural Publishing Inc; 2008: 405–434.
22. Node M, Seo T, Miyamoto A, Adachi A, Hashimoto M, Sakagami M. Frequency dynamics shift of vestibular evoked myogenic potentials in patients with endolymphatic hydrops. *Otol Neurotol.* 2005;26:1208–2113.
23. Seo T, Node M, Yukimasa A, Sakagami M. Furosemide loading vestibular evoked myogenic potential for unilateral Ménière's disease. *Otol Neurotol.* 2003;24:283–288.
24 Seo T, Node M, Miyamoto A, Yukimasa A, Terada T, Sakagami M. Three cases of cochleosaccular endolymphatic hydrops without vertigo revealed by furosemide-loading vestibular evoked myogenic potencial test. *Otol Neurolotol.* 2003;24: 807–811.
25. Rauch SD, Silveria MB, Zhou G, et al. Vestibular evoked myogenic potentials versus vestibular test battery in patients with Ménière's disease. *Otol Neurotol.* 2004;25(6):981–986.
26. Rauch SD, Zhou G, Kujawa SG, Guinan JJ, Herrmann BS. Vestibular evoked myogenic potentials show altered tuning in patients with Ménière's disease. *Otol Neurolotol.* 2004;25:333–338.
27. Janky K, Shepard NT. Vestibular evoked myogenic potential (VEMP) testing: normative threshold response curves and effects of age. *J Am Acad Audiol.* 2009; 20(8):514–522.
28. Lin MY, Timmer FCA, Oriel BS, et al. Vestibular evoked myogenic potential (VEMP) can detect asymptomatic saccular hydrops. *Laryngoscope.* 2006;116: 987–992.

29. Timmer FCA, Zhou G, Gainan JJ, Kujawa SG, Herrmann BS, Rauch SD. Vestibular evoked myogenic potential (VEMP) in patients with Ménière's disease with drop attacks. *Laryngoscope.* 2006;116:776–779.
30. Curthoys IS, Halmagyi GM. Vestibular compensation: clinical changes in vestibular function with time after unilateral vestibular loss. In: Herdman SJ, ed. *Vestibular Rehabilitation.* 3rd ed. Philadelphia, PA: FA Davis; 2007: 76–97.
31. Neuhauser H, Leopold M, von Brevern M, Arnold G, Lempert T. The interrelations of migraine, vertigo and migrainous vertigo. *Neurology.* 2001;56:436–441.

9

Other Diagnostic Tests

Michael J. Ruckenstein

Radiologic Studies

An MRI study with paramagnetic enhancement (eg, gadolinium) is, with very few exceptions, a required test in all patients suspected of having Ménière's disease.[1,2] The purpose of the MRI is to rule out lesions involving the VIIIth cranial nerve (most commonly an acoustic neuroma) and central lesions (eg, multiple sclerosis) that can mimic Ménière's disease (Fig 9–1). The performance of the MRI obviates the need to perform evoked potential audiometry (eg, ABR) for diagnostic purposes. If gadolinium-based enhancing agents cannot be administered to a patient, then an MRI series incorporating 3D fast imaging employing steady-state acquisition (FIESTA) can provide detailed imaging of the internal auditory canals and should serve as an adequate screen to rule out all but the smallest tumors (Fig 9–2). If the patient cannot undergo an MRI scan (eg, due to presence of an implant with magnetic properties), then a fine-cut CT of the temporal with intravenous contrast can be performed.

In children and young adults (<30 years old), a CT scan of the temporal bone without contrast also should be obtained to rule out labyrinthine dysmorphologies. Such congenital dysmorphologies would include enlarged vestibular aqueduct syndrome or incomplete partitions (eg, Mondini's dysplasia) (Figs 9–3 and 9–4).[3]

Serologic and Immunologic Testing

Some questions remain as to what constitutes an inclusive yet cost-effective serologic and immunologic testing evaluation in patients suspected of having Ménière's disease. The goal of such testing is to rule out potentially treatable disorders that mimic Ménière's disease. With regard to testing for infectious disorders, the current evidence supports performing a test for late secondary or tertiary syphilis in all patients with symptoms of Ménière's disease.[4]

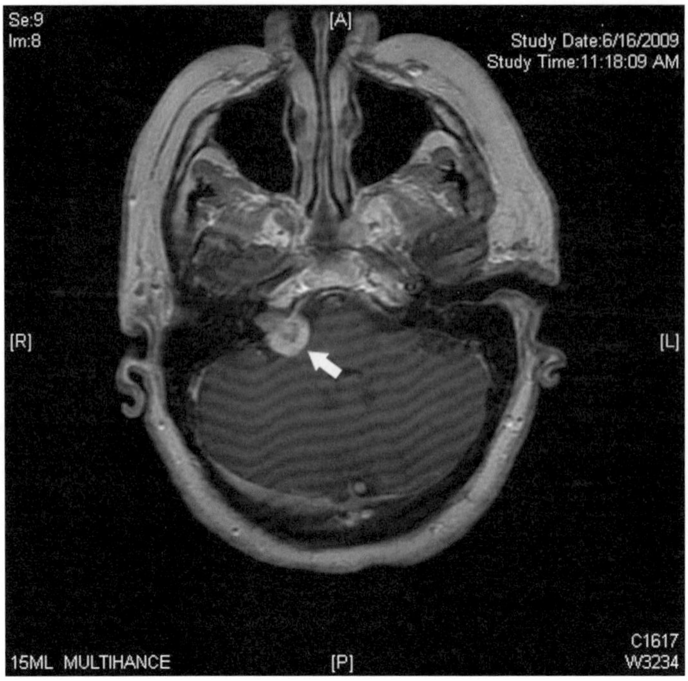

Fig 9–1. A T1-weighted axial MRI with gadolinium demonstrating an acoustic neuroma (*white arrow*).

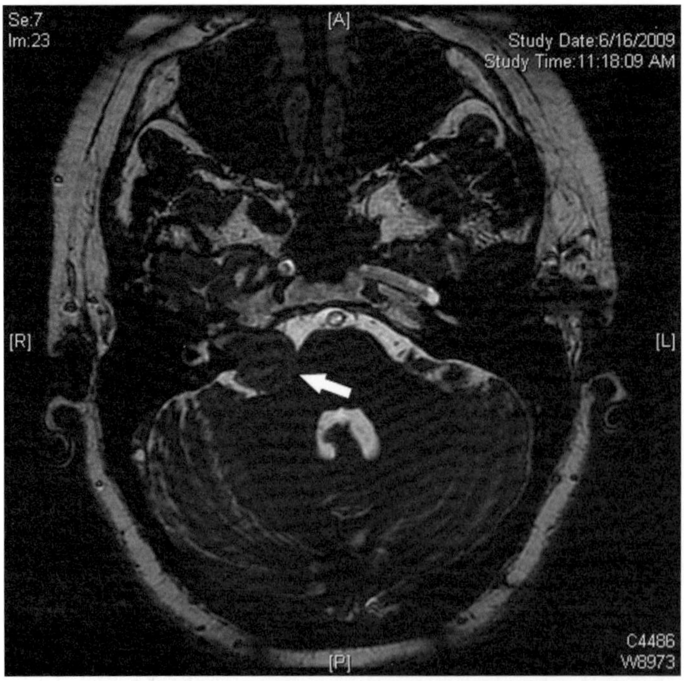

Fig 9–2. A FIESTA axial MRI scan demonstrating displacement of CSF in the internal auditory canal and cerebellopontine angle by an acoustic neuroma (*white arrow*).

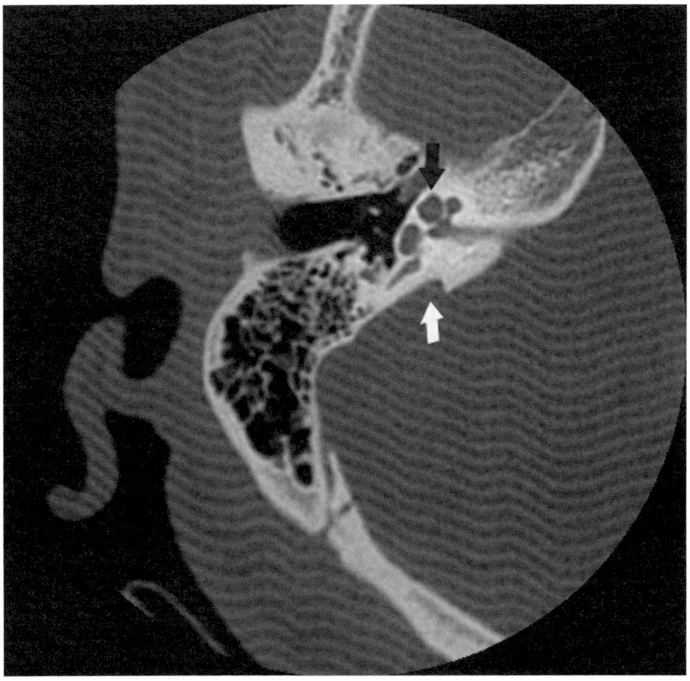

Fig 9–3. An axial CT scan demonstrating an enlarged vestibular aqueduct (*white arrow*) and an incomplete cochlear partition (*black arrow*).

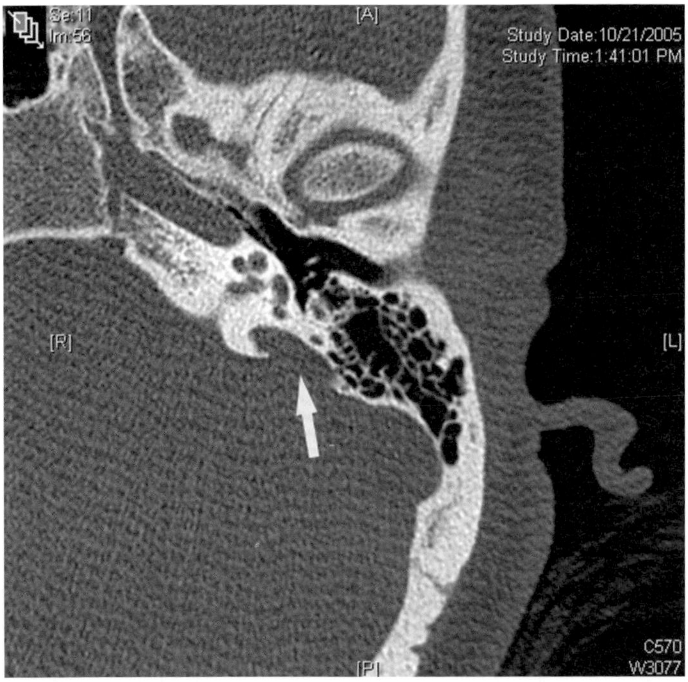

Fig 9–4. An axial CT scan demonstrating an enlarged vestibular aqueduct (*white arrow*).

Testing for syphilis needs to include evaluation for the *T. pallidum* antibody (eg, FTA-ABS, MHA-TP) to circumvent potential false negatives on the rapid plasma reagin (RPR). The test is easily performed and ubiquitously available and should be performed on all patients as part of their evaluation. Conversely, there is little to no evidence that the infection with the form of Lyme disease endemic in North America results in auditory or vestibular pathology.[4,5] In Europe, where a different genospecies of *B. burgorferi* is prevalent, testing for Lyme disease in patients suspected of having Ménière's disease is still recommended.[6]

Although there was, at one time, some enthusiasm for the hypothesis that Ménière's disease resulted from an autoimmune etiology,[7] as noted in Chapter 3 on pathophysiology, this does not appear to be the case. Nonetheless, there certainly are cases where autoimmune inner ear disease can present with symptoms similar to those found in Ménière's disease. Current evidence supports the use of a very minimal series of blood tests for immune/inflammatory processes in these patients.[8] A complete blood count (CBC), sedimentation rate (ESR), and C-reactive protein (CRP) tests are good screens for the presence of an inflammatory process. It would seem prudent to incorporate these general, easily performed, and inexpensive screening tests in patients suspected of having Ménière's disease. Elevations in antinuclear antibodies (ANAs) generally are associated with autoimmune diseases such as lupus and we did find them to be elevated in a significant number of patients with bilateral disease.[8] The significance of these elevations presently is unclear as the majority of these patients did not manifest any other evidence of autoimmune disease. Similarly, we have found elevations in antiphospholipid antibodies in patients with unilateral disease.[5,9] Elevations in antiphospholipid antibodies are associated with coagulopathic states. Therefore, it is attractive to hypothesize that, in some cases, symptoms of Ménière's disease might be the result of blood clots or emboli in the microcirculation of the inner ear. At present, this hypothesis cannot be confirmed. When it was first described, there was some evidence of association of the presence of an antibody to a 68-kD bovine inner ear antigen that also bound to the inducible form of heat shock protein-70.[10] However, further studies have not confirmed this association.[8,11–13]

In summary, a limited panel of serologic and immunologic tests can be recommended for patients undergoing a diagnostic workup for Ménière's disease:

- CBC
- ESR
- CRP
- MHA-TP or equivalent (eg, FTA-ABS)
- ANA
- Lyme serology (in Europe, but not North America)

References

1. Cueva RA. Auditory brainstem response versus magnetic resonance imaging for the evaluation of asymmetric sensorineural hearing loss. *Laryngoscope.* 2004; 114(10):1686–1692.
2. Ruckenstein MJ, Cueva RA, Morrison DH, Press G. A prospective study of ABR and MRI in the screening for vestibular schwannomas. *Am J Otol.* 1996;17(2): 317–320.

3. Berrettini S, Forli F, Bogazzi F, et al. Large vestibular aqueduct syndrome: audiological, radiological, clinical, and genetic features. *Am J Otolaryngol.* 2005;26(6):363–371.
4. Abuzeid WM, Ruckenstein MJ. Spirochetes in otology: are we testing for the right pathogens? *Otolaryngol Head Neck Surg.* 2008;138(1):107–109.
5. Ruckenstein MJ, Prasthoffer A, Bigelow DC, Von Feldt JM, Kolasinski SL. Immunologic and serologic testing in patients with Ménière's disease. *Otol Neurotol.* 2002;23(4):517–520; discussion 520–521.
6. Moscatello AL, Worden DL, Nadelman RB, Wormser G, Lucente F. Otolaryngologic aspects of Lyme disease. *Laryngoscope.* 1991;101(6 pt 1):592–595.
7. Ruckenstein MJ. Autoimmune inner ear disease. *Curr Opin Otolaryngol Head Neck Surg.* 2004;12(5):426–430.
8. Ruckenstein MJ, Prasthoffer A, Bigelow DC, Von Feldt JM, Kolasinski SL. Immunologic and serologic testing in patients with Ménière's disease. *Otol Neurotol.* 2002;23(4):517–520.
9. Mouadeb DA, Ruckenstein MJ. Antiphospholipid inner ear syndrome. *Laryngoscope.* 2005;115(5):879–883.
10. Gottschlich S, Billings PB, Keithley EM, Weisman MH, Harris JP. Assessment of serum antibodies in patients with rapidly progressive sensorineural hearing loss and Ménière's disease [see comment]. *Laryngoscope.* 1995;105(12 pt 1):1347–1352.
11. Rauch SD, Zurakowski D, Bloch DB, Bloch KJ. Anti-heat shock protein 70 antibodies in Ménière's disease. *Laryngoscope.* 2000;110(9):1516–1521.
12. Garcia Berrocal JR, Ramirez-Camacho R, Arellano B, Vargas JA. Validity of the Western blot immunoassay for heat shock protein-70 in associated and isolated immunorelated inner ear disease. *Laryngoscope.* 2002;112(2):304–309.
13. Riente L, Bongiorni F, Nacci A, et al. Antibodies to inner ear antigens in Ménière's disease. *Clin Exp Immunol.* 2004;135(1):159–163.

10

Medical Treatment of Ménière's Disease

Jessica Shen and Michael J. Ruckenstein

Introduction

The treatment of Ménière's disease remains both elusive and controversial. The most significant barrier to definitive treatment is a lack of understanding of its underlying etiology. A variety of therapeutic options have been studied with conflicting results. Although there is no cure for Ménière's disease, patients nevertheless are able to achieve significant symptom improvement. This chapter offers a critical, evidenced-based review of currently available options for medical treatment of Ménière's disease.

General Considerations

Any discussion on the treatment of Ménière's disease must incorporate an analysis of the placebo effect that characterizes many of the therapies associated with this disorder. Nicholas Torok was among the first researchers to formally document the nonspecific or placebo response exhibited by patients with Ménière's disease to a wide variety of therapies.[1] Torok reported that a 60% to 80% positive therapeutic response was exhibited to virtually any intervention in the short to intermediate term. These findings, which have since been confirmed by others,[2] and must be considered when analyzing studies of treatment of Ménière's disease.

What Is the Placebo Effect?

The placebo effect can be defined as a "specific, beneficial response elicited by the administration of a nonspecific or an inert intervention."[3] Two basic neurobiological mechanisms have been identified that are involved in mediating the placebo effect.[4] Expectation of cure is more commonly seen in situations involving conscious physiologic processes (eg, pain perception or motor function).[5] A conditioned response is the more dominant mechanism in unconscious physiologic processes (eg, immune modulation, hormone secretion).[5] Functional MRI, PET scanning, and EEG studies have provided important insights into the physiology of the placebo effect. Most important is the observation that placebos activate the *same neural pathways* as active treatments when exerting their physiologic effects. For example:

- In studies pertaining to pain, placebos were shown to activate endogenous opioid receptors in a pattern similar to that observed with the administration of true opiates.[6]
- Treatment of Parkinson's disease with placebo results in activation of nigrostriatal dopaminergic pathways.[5,7]
- Patients suffering from depression demonstrate similar neural response patterns when treated with placebo or active agents, particularly in the early stages of response.[5]

Thus, although the ingredients or interventions comprising the placebo itself may be nonspecific, the effects of the placebo intervention are very specific.[6] Active and placebo treatments have similar effects on neural activity resulting in an improvement in patients symptoms. Although we do not yet understand the pathophysiology of Ménière's disease, it would seem reasonable to assume that placebo treatments similarly are effecting a change in the neural processes mediating Ménière's disease.

Practical Implications of the Placebo Effect and Ménière's Disease

Based on the above discussion, the following conclusions must be considered when evaluating therapeutic trials of treatments for Ménière's disease:

- The high placebo response rate together with the fluctuating natural history of the disorder necessitate the inclusion of large numbers of patients in any placebo-controlled study of treatment efficacy in order to have sufficient power to overcome the "beta-error." This explains why so few high quality studies on treatment of Ménière's disease have been performed. The vast majority of studies of potential treatments for Ménière's disease are not placebo controlled.
- When evaluating short-term results (2 years or less) of uncontrolled studies, a therapeutic efficacy of 80% or less would be consistent with what can be expected from a placebo treatment
- When evaluating long-term results (5 years or more) of uncontrolled studies, a therapeutic efficacy of 60% or less would be consistent with what can be expected from a placebo treatment
- Although the effects of a placebo may be nonspecific, there is no question that they can benefit patients with Ménière's disease. Thus, it certainly is not inappro-

priate to utilize such nonspecific interventions as part of a therapeutic regimen. However, such treatments should:

- carry minimal risk of side effects
- carry a minimal financial burden
- not adversely affect quality of life
- be abandoned for more specific treatments with demonstrated therapeutic efficacy if the patient is not demonstrating a positive therapeutic response.

Dietary and Lifestyle Issues

Modifications in diet long have been considered a mainstay for the treatment of Ménière's disease. Dietary salt restriction has been a cornerstone of treatment for more than 70 years. [8–10] The theory behind salt restriction lies in the principle that Ménière's disease results from endolymphatic hydrops, or increased endolymphatic volume in the membranous labyrinth of the inner ear. Reducing salt intake reduces systemic water load, and theoretically helps to restore endolymph volume balance. As of yet, no study provides convincing evidence of salt restriction's role in Ménière's disease management.[2] Nonetheless, a low-salt diet continues to be widely encouraged. Most regimens call for a daily sodium intake of less than 2,000 milligrams, although some are more restrictive. A "common sense" low-salt diet is an example of a nonspecific or placebo intervention that meets all the criteria listed above. It can be instituted with no financial expenditure and should cause a minimal alteration in the quality of life of the patient. It has no adverse complications and is likely to have secondary cardiovascular benefits.

Some advocate an even more restrictive diet as outlined by Furstenberg.[8] In addition to restricting salt, this diet (and its various iterations) also severely restricts the intake of caffeine, chocolate, cheese, and alcohol. Many of these factors are known triggers for migraines, and as noted in Chapter 8, migrainous vertigo and Ménière's disease historically have been frequently confused. It is possible that these dietary restrictions did specifically benefit those patients who truly were suffering from episodes of migrainous vertigo. There also may be some nonspecific benefits. Today, when highly effective, minimally invasive treatment regimens are available to control vertigo, one has to question the merits of such a highly punitive and restrictive diet. Although objective confirmation is still lacking, it is reasonable to hypothesize that an intratympanic gentamicin injection carries less of an impact on a patient's quality of life than a diet restricted of chocolate, coffee, and wine!

Vestibular Suppressants

Vestibular suppressants and anti-emetic agents traditionally have been used to control acute vertigo attacks. All of these drugs have varying degrees of anticholinergic, anti-emetic, and sedative properties. Broadly, they can be divided into three classes: first generation (sedating) antihistamines, anticholinergics, and benzodiazepines.[11] Benzodiazepines have an additional beneficial anxiolytic effect. No strong data currently exist to support one abortive regime over another.

Diuretics

To date, diuretics are the most widely utilized pharmacologic agents for the treatment of Ménière's disease. The theoretical basis for their use is to diurese the inner ear, thus relieving the excess fluid volume associated with endolymphatic hydrops. Four main groups of diuretics have been investigated: thiazide diuretics, potassium sparing diuretics, loop diuretics, and carbonic anhydrase inhibitors. Thiazide diuretics (eg, hydrochlorthiazide) inhibit Na^+/Cl^- reabsorption the distal convoluted tubules of the nephron. Potassium sparing diuretics (eg, spironolactone, amiloride, triamterene) inhibit Na^+/K^+ exchange in nephron collecting ducts. Loop diuretics (eg, furosemide) inhibit the sodium-potassium-chloride cotransporter in the thick ascending limb of the loop of Henle. Carbonic anhydrase inhibitors (eg, acetazolamide) inhibit the transport of bicarbonate out of the proximal convoluted tubule into the interstitium, which leads to less sodium reabsorption at this site and therefore greater sodium, bicarbonate and water loss in the urine.

Strong evidence to support the benefit of diuretics is lacking. An early double-blind clinical trial by Klockhoff and Lindbolm comparing hydrochlorathiazide to placebo showed significant improvement in vertigo, quality of life, and hearing in the treatment group.[12] A reexamination of these data, however, revealed the study's design and data analyses were so seriously flawed that its conclusions had to be considered invalid.[2] These conclusions were echoed by a recent Cochrane review that concluded that there was insufficient evidence to support the efficacy of diuretics for the treatment of vertigo, hearing loss, tinnitus, or aural fullness in Ménière's disease.[13]

It is important to note that diuretics, although commonly used, are not benign. Side effects include renal and hepatic insufficiency, gastrointestinal discomfort, metabolic acidosis, nephrocalcinosis, paresthesias, hyperglycemia, hyperuricemia, hypokalemia, and hypochloremia. Despite the side effect profile, most consider diuretics to be a relatively safe option. Currently, the most commonly used diuretic for Ménière's disease is the combination of HCTZ and triamterene (Dyazide®). Utilization of this drug meets the criteria discussed above for the administration of a treatment with a nonspecific therapeutic benefit in that it is inexpensive, unlikely to adversely affect the overall quality of life of the patient, and carries a minimal risk of significant side effects. The beneficial effects of acetazolamide appear to be restricted to patients with a familial syndrome of vestibulocochlear degeneration associated with migraines.[14,15] The use of loop diuretics (eg, furosemide) for the treatment of Ménière's disease should be discouraged as they carry a greater risk of side effects.

Vasodilators

Vasodilators are another group of drugs that have been used extensively for the treatment of Ménière's disease, particularly in Europe.[16] They are presumed to function by improving the cochlear microcirculation.[17] Examples of vasodilators that have been used include niacin, isosorbide dinitrate, papaverine, histamine, and betahistine. Intravenous injections of histamine were, at one time quite popular, but largely have been discarded as treatment.[18] Betahistine, an oral congener of histamine, has thus far received the most research focus. As in the case of diuretics, evidence to support use of betahistine is controversial. Although some studies have demonstrated a beneficial effect of betahistine in patients with Ménière's disease,[19] the overall strength of such data is weak. A Cochrane review article regarding betahistine versus placebo in Ménière's disease found that, "no trial met the highest quality standard set by the review because of inadequate diagnostic criteria or methods, and none assessed the effect of betahistine on vertigo adequately."[20] The one study that had "good methods" showed no significant difference in tinnitus when comparing betahistine to placebo.

Some have suggested that the use of vasodilators Ménière's disease is counterintuitive.[1] Increasing blood flow to the stria vascularis theoretically should increase endolymph production, which in turn would exacerbate Ménière's disease. It also is seemingly illogical to treat patients with betahistine when antihistamines are used to abort acute attacks.

At present, there is no evidence that the efficacy of vasodilators in the treatment of Ménière's disease exceeds that exhibited by a placebo treatment. Nonetheless, a drug such as betahistine is inexpensive, unlikely to adversely affect a patient's quality of life, and carries a low risk of side effects. Therefore, like diuretics, betahistine's use can be justified as patients may benefit from its nonspecific therapeutic effects.

Hyposensitization Immunotherapy

As noted in a previous chapter, various hypotheses have been advanced to explain the etiology and pathogenesis of Ménière's disease. An immunologic basis for the disorder has been considered but, to date, no convincing evidence has been reported to suggest that it is an immune-mediated process.[21] In particular, there is no evidence of an allergic etiology for Ménière's disease. Hyposensitization immunotherapy has been suggested as a potential treatment for Ménière's disease for some time.[22,23] That said, there have been no controlled studies to evaluate the efficacy of this treatment. Furthermore, studies to date have not demonstrated a therapeutic response to hyposensitization therapy that exceeds what would be expected from a placebo treatment.[24] This treatment is time consuming, expensive, and carries some risk to the patient. Therefore, at this point in time, hyposensitization immunotherapy cannot be recommended as a treatment for Ménière's disease.

Pulse Pressure Therapy

As discussed in Chapter 3 on pathophysiology, it is not at all clear that the endolymphatic hydrops observed in temporal bones of patients with Ménière's disease is responsible for the symptoms associated with Ménière's disease. That said, treatments to improve or resolve the hydrops are still proposed with the hope that they will improve the symptoms of Ménière's disease. An example of such a treatment is the pulse pressure generator. This device was developed based on a theory developed by researchers in Sweden that hypothesized that external pressure changes can be transmitted to the perilymph leading to an alteration in inner ear fluid dynamics.[25,26] They propose that increasing perilymph fluid pressure will compress the endolymphatic fluid compartment forcing endolymph to drain out into the endolymphatic duct, thereby improving the hydrops. This led the investigators to develop a device (the Meniett) that applies pressure pulses to the middle ear via a tympanostomy tube.[27–29] Theoretically, these pressure pulses then are transmitted to the inner ear via the middle ear.

There is no evidence that the pulse waves generated by the Meniett are transmitted to the inner fluid compartments and affect their volumes. Application of the device did not result in any change in objective measures of auditory or vestibular function.[30] Much of the research performed with the device was conducted by the Meniett's inventors, thus creating potential conflicts of interest.[31] In fact, one of the papers touting the benefits of the Meniett was published as a "Letter to the Editor" with an advertisement for the Meniett device appearing on the same page.[27]

Recent independent uncontrolled and controlled studies are fairly consistent in demonstrating a therapeutic of 50% to 70% for follow-up periods of 18 months to 2 years.[32–34] It is not likely to be effective in patients who have failed a conservative surgical procedure.[31,35] One multicenter, placebo-controlled study did reveal a statistically significant improvement in AAO-HNS scale of functionality and a visual analog scale of vertigo in patients treated with the active device as opposed to a placebo device.[36] However, this study had a single endpoint, 2 months after initiation of treatment.

In summary, the Meniett is a relatively benign treatment, carrying complications associated with placement of middle ear ventilation tubes. However, it is expensive and unlikely to provide benefit that exceeds what would be expected from a placebo.

Conclusions

Currently, none of the available medical treatments appear to offer a therapeutic efficacy superior to a placebo. Thus, we do not have any treatments that specifically affect and modify the underlying disease process. That said, there are several interventions that, simply by invoking the placebo-effect, can benefit patients. These interventions—low salt diet, diuretics, betahistine—are inexpensive and carry low risk of side effects. Until the development of a more specific therapy, their use can be recommended as primary treatments for patients with Ménière's disease. The Meniett device and immunotherapy are expensive interventions that carry a therapeutic efficacy no better than that obtained with a placebo. In addition, immunotherapy imposes rare but significant risks on the patient. Thus, their general use in the treatment of patients with Ménière's disease is not supported by currently available data.

References

1. Torok N. Old and new in Ménière disease. *Laryngoscope.* 1977;87(11):1870–1877.
2. Ruckenstein MJ, Rutka JA, Hawke M. The treatment of Ménière's disease: Torok revisited. *Laryngoscope.* 1991; 101(2):211–218.
3. McQuay HJ, Moore RA. Placebo. *Postgrad Med J.* 2005;81(953):155–160.
4. Pacheco-Lopez G, Engler H, Niemi MB, Schedlowski M. Expectations and associations that heal: immunomodulatory placebo effects and its neurobiology. *Brain Behav Immun.* 2006;20(5):430–446.
5. Benedetti F, Mayberg HS, Wager TD, Stohler CS, Zubieta JK. Neurobiological mechanisms of the placebo effect. *J Neurosci.* 2005;25(45):10390–10402.
6. de la Fuente-Fernandez R, Schulzer M, Stoessl AJ. The placebo effect in neurological disorders. *Lancet Neurol.* 2002; 1(2):85–91.
7. De Beer L, Stokroos R, Kingma H. Intratympanic gentamicin therapy for intractable Ménière's disease. *Acta Otolaryngol (Stockh).* 2007;127(6):605–612.
8. Furstenberg AC, Lashmet FH, Lathrop F. Ménière's symptom complex: medical treatment. 1934. *Ann Otol Rhinol Laryngol.* 1992;101(1):20–31.
9. Santos PM, Hall RA, Snyder JM, Hughes LF, Dobie RA. Diuretic and diet effect on Ménière's disease evaluated by the 1985 Committee on Hearing and Equilibrium guidelines. *Otolaryngol Head Neck Surg.* 1993;109(4):680–689.
10. Jackson CG, Glasscock ME,3rd, Davis WE, Hughes GB, Sismanis A. Medical management of Ménière's disease. *Ann Otol Rhinol Laryngol.* 1981;90(2 pt 1): 142–147.
11. Straube A. Pharmacology of vertigo/ nystagmus/oscillopsia. *Curr Opin Neurol.* 2005;18(1):11–14.
12. Klockhoff I, Lindblom U. Ménière's disease and hydrochlorothiazide (Dichlotride)—a critical analysis of symptoms and therapeutic effects. *Acta Otolaryngol.* 1967;63(4):347–365.
13. Thirlwall AS, Kundu S. Diuretics for Ménière's disease or syndrome. *Cochrane Database Syst Rev.* 2006;3:CD003599.
14. Baloh RW, Winder A. Acetazolamide-responsive vestibulocerebellar syndrome: clinical and oculographic features. *Neurology.* 1991;41(3):429–433.
15. Baloh RW, Foster CA, Yue Q, Nelson SF. Familial migraine with vertigo and essential tremor. *Neurology.* 1996;46(2): 458–460.
16. Smith WK, Sankar V, Pfleiderer AG. A national survey amongst UK otolaryngologists regarding the treatment of Ménière's disease. *J Laryngol Otol.* 2005; 119(2):102–105.
17. Laurikainen EA, Miller JM, Quirk WS, et al. Betahistine-induced vascular effects in the rat cochlea. *Am J Otol.* 1993;14(1): 24–30.
18. Sheehy JL, Robinson JV, Bush JE. Intravenous histamine in otologic practice. Side effects in 2,347 administrations. *Arch Otolaryngol.* 1980;106(3):159–160.
19. Mira E, Guidetti G, Ghilardi L, et al. Betahistine dihydrochloride in the treatment of peripheral vestibular vertigo. *Eur Arch Otorhinolaryngol.* 2003;260(2):73–77.
20. James AL, Burton MJ. Betahistine for Ménière's disease or syndrome. *Cochrane Database Syst Rev.* 2001;(1)(1):CD001873.
21. Ruckenstein MJ. Immunologic aspects of Ménière's disease [Review] [45 refs]. *Am J Otolaryngol.* 1999;20(3):161–165.
22. Derebery MJ, Valenzuela S. Ménière's syndrome and allergy. *Otolaryngol Clin North Am.* 1992;25(1):213–224.
23. Derebery MJ. Allergic and immunologic aspects of Ménière's disease. *Otolaryngol Head Neck Surg.* 1996;114(3): 360–365.
24. Derebery MJ, Berliner KI. Allergy and Ménière's disease. *Curr Allergy Asthma Rep.* 2007;7(6):451–456.
25. Densert B, Densert O, Erlandsson B, Sheppard H. Transmission of complex

pressure waves through the perilymphatic fluid in cats. *Acta Otolaryngol.* 1986;102(5–6):403–409.
26. Densert B, Densert O, Erlandsson B, Sheppard H. Transmission of square wave pressure pulses through the perilymphatic fluid in cats. *Acta Otolaryngol.* 1986;102(3–4):186–193.
27. Densert B, Arlinger S, Odkvist LM. New technology to control symptoms in Ménière's disease. *Acta Otolaryngol.* 2000;120(5):672–674.
28. Densert B, Sass K. Control of symptoms in patients with Ménière's disease using middle ear pressure applications: two years follow-up. *Acta Otolaryngol.* 2001; 121(5):616–621.
29. Odkvist LM, Arlinger S, Billermark E, Densert B, Lindholm S, Wallqvist J. Effects of middle ear pressure changes on clinical symptoms in patients with Ménière's disease—a clinical multicentre placebo-controlled study. *Acta Otolaryngol Suppl.* 2000;543:99–101.
30. Stokroos R, Olvink MK, Hendrice N, Kingma H. Functional outcome of treatment of Ménière's disease with the Meniett pressure generator. *Acta Otolaryngol.* 2006;126(3):254–258.
31. Rajan GP, Din S, Atlas MD. Long-term effects of the Meniett device in Ménière's disease: the Western Australian experience. *J Laryngol Otol.* 2005;119(5):391–395.
32. Gates GA, Verrall A, Green JD Jr, Tucci DL, Telian SA. Meniett clinical trial: long-term follow-up. *Arch Otolaryngol Head Neck Surg.* 2006;132(12):1311–1316.
33. Mattox DE, Reichert M. Meniett device for Ménière's disease: use and compliance at 3 to 5 years. *Otol Neurotol.* 2008; 29(1):29–32.
34. Dornhoffer JL, King D. The effect of the Meniett device in patients with Ménière's disease: long-term results. *Otol Neurotol.* 2008;29(6):868–874.
35. Boudewyns AN, Wuyts FL, Hoppenbrouwers M, et al. Meniett therapy: rescue treatment in severe drug-resistant Ménière's disease? *Acta Otolaryngol.* 2005;125(12):1283–1289.
36. Thomsen J, Sass K, Odkvist L, Arlinger S. Local overpressure treatment reduces vestibular symptoms in patients with Ménière's disease: a clinical, randomized, multicenter, double-blind, placebo-controlled study. *Otol Neurotol.* 2005; 26(1):68–73.

11

Surgical Therapy in the Treatment of Ménière's Disease

Michael J. Ruckenstein, MD, and Marc A. Cohen, MD

The majority of patients who suffer from Ménière's disease can be managed successfully using a medical regimen while exploiting the natural course of the disease to remit and, ultimately, "burn out." It has been estimated that approximately 10% of patients with Ménière's disease require a surgical intervention.[1,2] When evaluating the reported outcomes for the wide variety of surgical interventions available for Ménière's disease, it is important to consider the following issues.

1. A plethora of surgical treatments have been described for Ménière's disease. Although some of the interventions are of historical interest, it is important for the practitioner to understand the implication of having this wide variety of procedures listed in the armamentarium. The diversity of treatments utilized in the past, including obsolete interventions such as cochlear dialysis, cryosurgery, ultrasonic radiation, and cochleosacculotomy, are a testament to our inability to derive a definitively effective surgical treatment. Thus the old adage, "if there are multiple ways to treat a disease, there is no good one."
2. The natural course of Ménière's disease provides a major confounding factor when evaluating treatment efficacy. Longitudinal studies have shown that from the time of presentation, approximately 70 to

80% of patients are free of symptoms at greater than 7 years regardless of whether there has been an intervention or not.[3–5] In his sentinel paper, Nicholas Torok reviewed 834 publications from 1951 to 1975 that reported on a wide range of treatment regimens.[6] He noted that, regardless of which treatment regimen was employed, recovery was seen in 60 to 80%, with 20 to 30% of patients improving, and 10 to 25% of patients being considered treatment failures. The results of this review, which was a precursor to our current "evidence-based" method of analysis, have been reaffirmed by others.[7]

3. Inclusion criteria for entry into a study about a particular intervention vary significantly. Although many studies state that patients who undergo surgery have "failed medical therapy" the definition of what constitutes a medical failure is not established. In part, this is due to a variable tolerance amongst patients for episodes of vertigo. Although one patient may consider one vertigo spell per month to be tolerable, another might find it to be an oppressive burden. The surgeon's bias must also be considered. Some centers and surgeons are much more likely to recommend a surgical intervention early on in the course of disease, whereas others take a much more conservative approach in selecting a particular therapy. The reasons for this are many and need not be explored here. That said, these different approaches do have significant implications in terms of data analysis. Given the natural course of the disease, a result of a surgical intervention given to a patient early in his or her course of illness will depend both on the efficacy of the procedure *and* the natural tendency of the disease to go into remission. Conversely, a patient who continues to have intractable vertigo despite multiple medical interventions extended over a more prolonged period of time is likely to have a more aggressive variant of disease. The efficacy of a surgical intervention provided to just this group of patients with more aggressive disease will be negatively impacted due to the inclusion criteria. In fact, patients with poorer disability ratings as per the AAO-HNS criterion have worse outcomes following surgical intervention.[8] Therefore, those requiring intervention the most are the least likely to derive benefit.
4. When comparing results derived from different studies, it is important for clinicians to note that investigators use diverse vestibular and hearing outcome measures for varying amounts of time, often leading to divergent conclusions with the same data set. Adequate adherence to AAO-HNS reporting criterion has been noted in only 50% of publications evaluating response to therapy in Ménière's disease.[9] Success as per the analysis of one author may be a failure to another.

With all these factors in mind, we can now embark on an analysis of the surgical literature. Surgical therapy for incapacitating vertiginous symptoms may be categorized as either hearing sparing or hearing ablative. With the advent of minimally invasive procedures, they can also be classified based on their degree of invasiveness and potential complications.

Cochlear Function Sparing Intervention

Intratympanic Therapies

The past two decades have seen an increase in interest in the use of intratympanic therapies to apply a therapeutic agent directly to the inner ear. This approach is attractive as it allows high doses of a therapeutic drug to access the inner ear rapidly and directly, avoiding delays and potential toxicities associated with systemic administration. Issues pertaining to intratympanic administration include permeability of a particular substance through the round window, distribution of the substance through the cochlea, and site of lesion within the cochlea. Permeability of a substance through the round window is dependent on its molecular weight and other physical characteristics.[10] Once through the round window, the majority of the agent will be concentrated at the basal turn of the cochlea and will not be distributed evenly along the length of the cochlea.[11] Once in the cochlea, the agent will have access to structures in contact with perilymph. Thus, if the site of lesion are in the stria vascularis or the cochlear nerve fibers, then intratympanic therapy would be expected to be less effective.

Despite these issues, the area of intratympanic therapy is an exciting one that is still in its infancy. With regard to Ménière's disease, there are currently two agents that are in clinical use; corticosteroids (mainly dexamethasone) and aminoglycosides (mainly gentamicin).

Intratympanic Corticosteroids

The use of corticosteroids for the treatment of Ménière's disease was prompted by the theory that the disorder may be immune mediated.[12] Studies have shown corticosteroids to be permeable through the round window membrane.[13] Although methylprednisolone appears to be the corticosteroid with the greatest round window permeability, dexamethasone has been used in the majority of clinical studies as the patient better tolerates its formulation.

At the time of publication, we could identify five studies published in the English language peer-reviewed literature.[14–18]

These five studies were diverse in terms of their designs and all reported results after short follow-up periods. Two of these studies were randomized double-blind placebo-controlled trials; however, one of these studies reported a follow-up of only 1 month. The other three were prospective or retrospective noncontrolled case series. All studies involved the administration of multiple doses of dexamethasone. These studies are summarized in Table 11–1. No significant complications including no evidence of ototoxicity were noted with this treatment.

The diverse study design and the short-term follow-up periods make it difficult to draw any strong conclusions about intratympanic dexamethasone treatment for Ménière's disease.

Table 11-1. Summary of Studies Using Intratympanic Dexamethasone

Study	*n*	*Design*	*Controlled*	*Dose*	*Follow-up*	*Outcome*
Boleas-Aguirre[14]	96	Retrospective	No	12 mg/mL given at variable intervals	2 years	70% did not opt for further treatment with an alternate regimen
Garduno-Anaya[16]	22	Prospective randomized, double blind	Placebo controlled	4 mg/mL injections given on 5 consecutive days	2 years	82% had total or substantial vertigo control vs. 52% in the placebo group
Barrs[18]	34	Retrospective case series	No	10 mg/mL QWeek × 4 weeks	2 years	42% had complete control using a multiple dosing regimen
Sennaroglu[15]	24	Prospective case series	No	Drops administered through a ventilation tube daily × 3 months	18 months	72% had complete or substantial vertigo control
Silverstein[17]	20	Prospective randomized, double blind	Placebo controlled	8 mg/mL in hyaluronic acid × 3 consecutive days	1 month	No difference between control and placebo treatment

Based on the data that are currently available, it would seem reasonable to conclude that:

1. Intratympanic dexamethasone represents a well-tolerated, low morbidity procedure.
2. Vertigo control rates for dexamethasone are approximately equivalent to what one would expect from a placebo.
3. Dosing regimens should include multiple injections, with repeat injections at times of recurrence.

Intratympanic Aminoglycosides

Aminoglycosides have long been known to have variable degrees of vestibulotoxic and cochleotoxic effects.[19] Of the aminoglycosides, streptomycin and gentamicin demonstrate a greater degree of vestibulotoxicity versus cochleotoxicity. Shuckneckt was the first to try to take advantage of these pharmacologic properties by administering intratympanic streptomycin in an effort to obtain vestibular ablation while preserving hearing.[20] Although streptomycin is selectively vestibulotoxic, this intervention created sensorineural hearing loss in all five patients treated. Despite this early failure in hearing preservation, interest in using intratympanic aminoglycosides persisted. A considerable experience developed in Europe in the 1970s and 1980s with intratympanic gentamicin.[21–22] The treatment was brought to North America by Nedzelski and his colleagues,[23] and since that time a wealth of clinical and basic science papers have been published on the subject. A number of studies have reported long-term follow-up data for patients 5 years or more posttreatment.[24–26]

When evaluating studies pertaining to gentamicin inner ear perfusion, there are several issues that must be considered.

1. Desired therapeutic outcome. The overall treatment goal of using this treatment is to eliminate vertigo while preserving hearing. Yet, how is this goal best achieved? Should one strive for a complete unilateral vestibular ablation, so that the treatment effect is similar to that achieved with a vestibular nerve section or labyrinthectomy? This would seem to be a reasonable goal, but what if achieving this goal comes at the risk of increased hearing loss?
2. Dosing regimen. Different dosing regimens have been advocated so as to attempt to maximize vertigo control while minimizing the complication of hearing loss. These treatment strategies have included:
   a. Continuous dosing administered with a minipump, Merocel sponge, or similar device positioned next to the round window membrane (eg, ref. 27).
   b. Multiple daily doses (typically 3 doses per day for 4 consecutive days) administered through a catheter placed into the middle ear with a port fixed to auricle allowing for repeated injections (eg, ref. 28).
   c. Doses given weekly through a myringotomy or ventilation tube for 3 to 4 consecutive weeks (eg, ref. 29).
   d. Doses given at a regular interval until some evidence of an effect of the drug is present (eg, increased

hearing loss, evidence of a new onset peripheral vestibular loss on exam or testing) (eg, ref. 30).
   e. Single dose therapy with a repeat dose only with recurrence or persistence of vertigo (eg, ref. 31).
3. Some patients are genetically susceptible to ototoxicity with the use of aminoglycosides.[32,33] That said, an analysis of patients who suffered severe cochlear and vestibular loss during the course of treatment failed to reveal presence of this mutation in these patients.[34] Similarly, some patients may be resistant to the drugs effects.
4. The ototoxic effects of gentamicin do not occur immediately, but, rather, are delayed while the drug is metabolized. The delay in effect can be as long as 1 to 2 weeks. Thus, if a continuous dose regimen is being used, then titration to patients' symptoms or evidence of a vestibular loss may result in "overshooting" the desirable dose.
5. Evaluation of hearing loss in patients having undergone gentamicin treatment can be complicated by the natural course of the disease. Hearing will fluctuate and ultimately decline as part of the disease process itself. Salt et al have evaluated distribution of gentamicin throughout the cochlea using a predictive computer model.[35] Findings of this study indicate that use of either single dose treatments or treatments that are widely spaced apart are unlikely to produce concentrations sufficient to alter hearing. Furthermore, hearing fluctuations noted during such treatment regimens are likely due to the natural course of the disease and not the gentamicin treatments.

With these issues in mind, an analysis of the results of the various methods of intratympanic gentamicin is possible. This analysis is facilitated by two excellent meta-analyses that have carefully evaluated this form of treatment.[36,37] Chia et al performed a meta-analysis evaluating 27 studies with 980 patients whereas Cohen-Kerem et al's meta-analysis evaluated 15 publications with treatment of 627 patients. Ten of the 15 manuscripts evaluated by Cohen-Kerem et al were included in Chia et al's study. The results of Chia et al's study are summarized in Table 11–2. These data demonstrate that total vertigo control can be obtained in 70 to 80% of patients and total or substantial vertigo control is seen in better than 90% of patients. Patients undergoing low-dose therapy (single injection repeated only with recurrent symptoms) had significantly inferior vertigo control and titration therapy (treatment stopped with evidence of gentamicin effect) demonstrated significantly better vertigo control, when compared to other treatment methods. These results are echoed in Cohen-Kerem et al's analysis that showed approximately 93% of patients had complete or substantial vertigo control.[37] This meta-analysis did not find a statistical or clinical difference in vertigo control when it divided studies based on whether injection number was fixed or titrated to the patients' symptoms. There was a trend toward better vertigo control (92%) in patients whose vestibular function tests indicated a complete vestibular ablation when compared to patients who obtained a partial vestibular ablation (75%).[36]

The complication of hearing loss has always been a concern when administering gentamicin. As noted above, it

Table 11–2. Summary of Results of Meta-Analysis[36]

	Complete vertigo control (%)	Complete + substantial vertigo control (%)	Incidence of increased hearing loss (%)
Overall	76	90	25
Titration	81	96	24
Low Dose	67	87	24
Multiple Daily	76	91	35
Weekly	75	89	13
Continuous	71	89	24

is somewhat difficult to determine if changes in hearing are caused by gentamicin or the natural course of disease. The incidence of increased hearing loss ranged from 13% (weekly) to 35% (multiple daily) with the majority of treatment regimens eliciting an incidence of approximately 25% (see Table 11–2).[36] Although the incidence of increased hearing loss would seem to be substantial, analysis of the magnitude of hearing loss indicated that it is small, with a trend towards less hearing loss (0.02 dB) in the titration group compared to the fixed intervention (5.4 dB).[37] The incidence of increased hearing loss tended to be greater in patients who obtained a complete vestibular ablation (37%) when compared to those who demonstrated a partial vestibular loss (25%).

In summary, the following conclusions may be drawn from the data presented above regarding intratympanic gentamicin treatments.

1. Intratympanic gentamicin offers complete or substantial vertigo control in better than 90% of patients for periods of 2 to 5 years or more.
2. An increase in hearing loss is noted in approximately 25% of patients; however, the magnitude of this hearing loss is small.
3. Titration strategies, in which the injections are discontinued with evidence of an effect of the drug (new onset hearing loss or vestibular loss), appear to maximize vertigo control.
4. Vertigo control appears to be better in patients who obtain a complete vestibular ablation as exhibited by balance function testing.
5. Vertigo control rates obtained by intratympanic gentamicin treatment exceed those expected from placebo.

Endolymphatic Sac Surgery

First described in 1927 by Portmann,[38] 11 years prior to identification of the pathologic hallmark of Ménière's disease —endolymphatic hydrops,[7] endolymphatic sac surgery remains a popular surgical intervention for Ménière's disease.[39] Since its popularization in the 1960s, it has been one of the most controversial in neurotology. In fact, Schuknecht included endolymphatic shunt surgery as one of his "myths of neurotology."[40] Both its adherents and detractors approach endolympatic sac surgery with almost a religious fervor! One of the most frequent questions encountered by the senior author during his presentations on Ménière's disease is, "Do you *believe* in endolymphatic sac surgery?" Fortunately, the many publications that have been contributed to the literature allow for a dispassionate assessment of the efficacy of endolympathic sac surgery.

Surgeries involving the endolymphatic sac are broadly divided into 4 types: (1) endolymphatic sac incision, (2) endolymphatic subarachnoid shunting, (3) endolymphatic mastoid shunting, and (4) endolymphatic decompression. The evolution of surgeries involving the endolymphatic sac is noteworthy as Portmann's initial technique involved decompression, quite similar to both Shambaugh's technique in 1969 as well as the more recent wide posterior fossa decompression endolymphatic sac vein decompression technique.[38,41–43] House popularized the endolymphatic subarachnoid shunt.[44] This method was altered further with the description of an endolymphatic mastoid shunt, which reduced the risk of intracranial and hearing complications.[45] In the creation of an endolymphatic mastoid shunt, authors have described incision and opening of the sac or incision and placement of a Silastic sheet, tubing, or one-way valve.[46–48]

A critical review of the extensive reports pertaining to the efficacy of endolymphatic sac surgery allows the following conclusions to be made.

1. Approximately 80 to 90% of patients undergoing endolymphatic sac surgery have total or substantial vertigo control at 2 years after surgery. With an increasing period of follow-up, the chance of a favorable therapeutic result declines. At 5 years postsurgery, approximately 60% of patients have a total or substantial vertigo control. Vertigo control further declines at 10-year follow-up. It must be emphasized that these data pertain to the results of a single surgical intervention. Some studies incorporate results of primary and subsequent revision surgeries into a single data pool. Given the potential placebo response to this surgery, this approach to analysis inflates the apparent benefit. Conversely, other authors confine their outcome measure to *total* vertigo control. This more rigid criterion of surgical success diminishes the apparent benefit.[42,49–60]
2. The therapeutic results of the various surgical modifications to endolymphatic sac surgery described above are essentially equivalent.
3. Regardless of the method used, endolymphatic sac surgery is of low risk with less than 1% of complete sensorineural.[49,61] Rare complications include CSF leak, facial paralysis, vertigo, and wound infection.

Significant controversy regarding the efficacy of endolymphatic sac procedures followed the publication of the randomized, double-blind, "Danish Sham Surgery" study by Thomsen et al.[62–65] This study evaluated 30 patients with

Ménière's disease refractory to medical treatment; 15 of whom were randomized into the "active" surgical group undergoing endolymphatic mastoid shunt with the control group of 15 patients undergoing a "placebo" mastoidectomy. The primary outcome measure was vertigo control. Secondary outcome measures included changes in audiometric data, changes in patients' assessments of symptoms, and patient and surgeon evaluation of efficacy of the procedure (both patient and surgeon were blinded as to the specific surgery performed).

Both sac surgery and mastoidectomy groups demonstrated a reduction in vertigo, however, there was no difference in the level of vertigo control when the sac surgery and mastoidectomy groups were compared. These findings were consistent at 1, 3, 6, and 9-year follow-up evaluations. The conclusion drawn from the study was that endolymphatic sac surgery was no better than a placebo procedure in controlling vertigo in patients with Ménière's disease.

Given the pervasive use of endolymphatic sac surgery in the treatment of Ménière's disease, it is not surprising that these publications provoked both controversy and criticism. The majority of the criticism has been leveled at the interpretation of the data at the 1-year follow-up.[66,67] A recent reassessment of the original data by Welling et al, did show statistical differences between groups when comparing patient diary assessments in postoperative dizziness and aural pressure.[67] However, it must be pointed out that these authors did not have access to the original raw data, but rather derived the data from the figures published in the first publication.

Current readers of the Danish Sham Study and its associated critiques, benefit from a broader perspective that only time can afford. What have we learned from this study?

1. Both patients in the active (sac) surgery and placebo (mastoidectomy) arms of the study demonstrate a dramatic reduction in vertigo. That a placebo surgery can result in a resolution of symptoms of vertigo in close to 70% of patients is truly a remarkable finding. Yet, the debate over the meaning of the study has focused on possible differences in symptom control rates *between* groups that are negligible in magnitude when compared to overall response rate in *both* groups. When reviewing the literature on this subject, one cannot help but feel that during this debate, the proverbial forest was lost for the trees. Understanding why the physical symptoms of Ménière's disease demonstrate such a dramatic response to nonspecific or placebo therapy may well hold the key to understanding the disorder itself. In retrospect, one would have hoped that the Danish Sham Study would have galvanized research into the fundamental pathophysiologic mechanisms governing Ménière's disease, with particular emphasis on the central nervous system's ability to mitigate the disease as exhibited by the demonstrated placebo effect. Unfortunately, this has not proven to be the case.
2. Debate over the significance of the differences in vertigo control between sac and mastoidectomy procedures likely will never be resolved. Nor does it have to be resolved. At subsequent follow-up periods, there

is no difference in the vertigo control rates—in fact, the placebo arms seems to fair somewhat better! Long-term vertigo control rates are what are of interest to both the patient and the surgeon. These rates have been well established from noncontrolled studies as described above.
3. The premature unblinding of the study due to Denmark's acceptance of the Helsinki Declaration on medical ethics contributed to a small study population and a lack of statistical power. The resulting beta-error is likely significant when interpreting the results reported at 1-year follow-up. However, using the same logic, one must also conclude that the similarity in the long-term results of the 2 groups indicates that an extremely large number of patients would have to be included in a study in order to demonstrate any significant difference in vertigo control rates.

Vestibular Nerve Section

Sectioning of the vestibular nerve offers a method of preservation of auditory function while eliminating the peripheral afferent input from the pathologic inner ear. For many years, it was the treatment of choice for hearing preservation and vertigo control for patients with Ménière's disease. It is still the gold standard against which any intervention purporting to offer similar benefits must compare itself.

In 1898, the first vestibular nerve section was performed by Fedor Krause, a German neurosurgeon.[68] Walter Dandy receives credit for the earliest series of vestibular neurectomy for vertigo using the suboccipital approach.[68,69] Interest in the procedure waned in the middle portion of the 20th century until House resurrected it in the 1960s with his middle fossa approach with microscopic visualization for vestibular nerve section.[70] Since that time the procedure has been performed using various techniques that can be summarized as follows.

1. The middle fossa approach. As described by House, the internal auditory canal is identified on the floor of the internal auditory canal via a temporal craniotomy. Fisch modified the approach my removing portions of the superolateral temporal bone to minimize temporal lobe retraction.[71] The approach is highly efficacious, with long-term vertigo control rates of approximately 95% being reported in multiple studies.[71–75] Hearing is preserved in a similar percentage of patients. Despite its therapeutic efficacy, the middle fossa approach is technically difficult and can result in inadvertent entry into the labyrinth. It was not favored in older patients due to the risk of central complications from temporal lobe retraction. In addition, the position of the facial nerve makes it more susceptible to trauma in this approach—with the incidence of temporary facial paralysis being approximately 5 to 10%. The technical challenges posed by this procedure resulted in the development of alternative techniques.
2. The retrolabyrinthine approach. In 1978, in an attempt to minimize intracranial complications and to simplify the procedure, Silverstein

advocated for the retrolabyrinthine approach.[76] This transmastoid approach involved approaching the nerve in the posterior fossa by removing the bone between the sigmoid sinus posteriorly and the facial nerve and vestibular labyrinth anteriorly. The VIIIth cranial nerve is identified and the superiorly positioned vestibular nerve is separated from the inferiorly placed cochlear nerve along a cleavage plane that must be estimated by the surgeon. The approach is familiar to most otologists and carries less risk to the labyrinth, facial nerve, and brain when compared to the middle fossa approach. However, it does not quite achieve the vertigo control rates reported using the middle fossa approach, with 80 to 90% of patients reporting complete or substantial vertigo control. The main reason for the somewhat inferior vertigo control rates is likely most attributable to the fact the nerve is transected prior to it separating from the cochlear nerve in the internal auditory canal. Thus, the surgeon must estimate the cleavage plane between the vestibular and cochlear nerves based on differences in hue of the two nerves or the position of a small vessel or the nervus intermedius that may course along the cleavage plane. In addition, the approach can provide restricted visualization of the posterior fossa, particularly in cases of a sclerotic mastoid, high riding jugular bulb, and/or anterior sigmoid sinus. Although complications are generally very low in this procedure, it does carry a higher risk of CSF leak of up to 10%.[76–79] The inferior vertigo control rate and the higher risk of CSF leak prompted some surgeons to further modify the approach.

3. The retrosigmoid and the retrosigmoid-internal auditory canal (RS-IAC) approaches. The retrosigmoid (suboccipital) approach is the "workhorse" approach for neurosurgeons accessing the posterior fossa. The VIIIth cranial nerve can easily be identified through this approach, the vestibular and cochlear nerves separated along the cleavage plane as described above in the retrolabyrinthine approach, and the vestibular nerve cut. Using the suboccipital approach avoids any restriction of visualization associated with the retrolabyrinthine approach. The complication of CSF leak is rare but headaches can be an issue in approximately 5% of patients. Complete or substantial control of vertigo is observed in 85 to 95% of patients.[80–82]

The retrosigmoid-internal auditory canal (RS-IAC) approach was offered as a means to improve vertigo control by identifying sectioning the vestibular nerve within the internal auditory canal, thus eliminating the need to estimate a cleavage plane between the vestibular and cochlear nerves.[83] Vertigo control rates of better than 95% are reported for this procedure.[77,84] The most prevalent complication is headache, which occurred at a rate of 36% in Silverstein's original series. This headache rate can be mitigated by the performance of a cranioplasty and by minimizing bone dust entering the CSF during drilling of the IAC, but postoperative headaches will still be reported in approximately 10% of patients. Temporary facial weakness and CSF leak are seen in less than 5% of patients. Some decrement in hearing can be detected in 25 to 40% of patients but total hearing loss is a rare complication. The retrosigmoid retrolabyrinthine approach allows for transection of the vestibular nerve in either the internal auditory canal or cerebellopontine angle.[77,83] The combined approach is technically easier and allows for less brain retraction and thus, less intracranial complications. Also of note with respect to procedures for vestibular neurectomy is the translabyrinthine vestibular nerve section, which is discussed later in this chapter.

In summary, vestibular nerve section offers an excellent method of controlling vertigo while preserving hearing. A retrosigmoid approach offers a straightforward method for most surgeons to access and section the vestibular nerve. Identifying the vestibular nerve in the internal auditory canal likely results in a more complete nerve section and this may translate in better vertigo control rates, although this claim has yet to be substantiated. Drilling out the IAC may result is a slightly greater incidence of CSF leak, hearing loss, headache, and facial paralysis. In experienced hands, a retrolabyrinthine approach can be utilized but it offers a more limited exposure and a higher rate of CSF leak than the retrosigmoid approach. The middle fossa approach is rarely advocated today for the purpose of vestibular nerve section due its increased technical difficulties and higher risk of complications.

Labyrinthectomy

Labyrinthectomy is a tried and true procedure for the treatment of Ménière's disease in patients without serviceable hearing in the affected ear. A properly performed transmastoid labyrinthectomy ensures the complete ablation of the vestibular end organ.[85] A transcanal approach where instruments of various shapes and angles were passed through the oval window to remove vestibular epithelium was popular for a time but is rarely performed today. Various other techniques have been advanced to ablate the labyrinth including the application of hypertonic saline, ultrasound, and cryoprobes.[86–88] However, none of these techniques have gained wide acceptance.

Labyrinthectomy should control vertigo in upward of 95% of cases. Failure to control vertigo might result from an incomplete labyrinthectomy (eg, failing to access the posterior canal ampulla), bilateral disease, or superimposed migrainous vertigo in a patient with Ménière's disease. Significant postoperative disequilibrium is seen in the majority of cases, and this is usually well addressed with the prompt institution of vestibular rehabilitation physical therapy.

Some surgeons have proposed that a translabyrinthine nerve section, a technique in which the vestibular nerve is accessed at the internal auditory canal following labyrinthectomy, may lead to better control of vestibular symptoms. This was suggested after noting the presence of a traumatic neuroma in the vestibule following labyrinthectomy as a result of leaving Scarpa's ganglion, which may lead to postoperative vestibulopathy.[89] Langman and Lindeman noted that there were no significant differences in the incidence of vertigo when comparing patients treated with transmastoid labyrinthectomy or translabyrinthine vestibular nerve section.[90] De La Cruz et al also compared transmastoid labyrinthectomy and translabyrinthine vestibular nerve section and found no difference in vertigo control rates in the 2 groups.[91] Therefore, it appears that transmastoid labyrinthectomy and translabyrinthine vestibular nerve section offer similar rates of vertigo control and, therefore, that the morbidity of intracranial surgery with translabyrinthine vestibular nerve section is not indicated.

Adjunct Therapy

As is the case with the treatment of any vestibulopathy, the importance of either primary or posttreatment vestibular rehabilitation and physical therapy must be emphasized. This is especially the case following acute decompensation or any intervention that results in vestibular obliteration. Patients with acute changes will invariably have an easier transition if vestibular rehabilitation is integrated earlier in the process.

The natural progression and treatment of Ménière's disease often leads to severe sensorineural hearing loss and, in some cases, is present in both ears. In those few individuals that develop these manifestations, some authors have advocated for cochlear implantation. In one recent publication by Lustig et al, the authors report excellent outcomes for those patients undergoing cochlear implantation, even in those patients that had undergone labyrinthectomy.[92] At this time, cochlear implantation seems to be a valuable adjunct in the management of Ménière's disease.

Conclusions

The data presented above justify the following conclusions:

1. In patients with unilateral Ménière's disease who fail medical therapy, intratympanic gentamicin administered using a titration technique should be the treatment of first choice. It offers long-term vertigo control rates of better than 85%, with minimal risk to hearing. Imbalance after gentamicin treatment is usually transient and can be treated effectively with vestibular rehabilitation physical therapy. The procedure is performed in an outpatient setting avoiding the expenses associated with hospital admission and the risks of an open surgical procedure.
2. Patients who are resistant to intratympanic gentamicin may benefit from a middle ear exploration to eliminate any anatomic obstructions that prevent the drug from accessing the round window membrane. In that small subset of patients whose vertigo recurs quickly despite gentamicin treatment, a more aggressive surgical treatment is indicated. A vestibular nerve section provides excellent vertigo control rates patients with serviceable hearing. A labyrinthectomy is preferred in patients without serviceable hearing in the affected ear as it

carries slightly less risk of complications (CSF leak, headache) than a nerve section. In addition, a labyrinthectomy preserves the possibility of rehabilitation with a cochlear implant should this be required.

3. Intratympanic dexamethasone and endolymphatic sac surgery do provide some benefits to patients. In both cases, the beneficial effects are likely mediated through a "nonspecific" or "placebo" mechanism. They both carry low risk, with dexamethasone being particularly benign. Intratympanic dexamethasone is performed in an outpatient setting avoiding the expenses associated with hospital admission and the risks of an open surgical procedure. However, both procedures offer inferior long-term vertigo control rates when compared to other treatment options (40 to 60%). Thus, their use should be reserved for patients who are very risk averse or who have bilateral disease and cannot undergo a vestibuloablative therapy.
4. Surgical results will only be as good as surgical indications. It is critical that a patient being considered for a vestibuloablative therapy carry a diagnosis of Ménière's disease. For example, migrainous vertigo can be confused with Ménière's disease but will not respond to an ablative treatment.

References

1. Glasscock GE, Gulya AJ, Pensak ML, et al. Medical and surgical management of Ménière's disease. *Am J Otol.* 1984;5:536–542.
2. Schessel DA, Minor LB, Nedzelski, J. Ménière's disease and other peripheral vestibular disorders. In Cummings CW, Flint PW, Haughey BH, et al, eds. *Cummings Otolaryngology Head and Neck Surgery.* 4th ed. St Louis, MO: Elsevier Mosby; 2005, 2672–2705.
3. Silverstein H, Smoutha E, Jones R. Natural history vs. surgery for Ménière's disease. *Otolaryngol Head Neck Surg.* 1989;1:6–16.
4. Quaranta A, Marini F, Sallustio V. Long-term outcome of Ménière disease: endolymphatic mastoid shunt versus natural history. *Audiol Neurotol.* 1998;3:54–60.
5. Green JD Jr, Blum DJ, Harner SG. Longitudinal follow-up of patients with Ménière's disease. *Otolaryngol Head Neck Surg.* 1991;104:783–788.
6. Torok N. Old and new in Ménière's disease. *Laryngoscope.* 1977;87:1870–1877.
7. Ruckenstein MJ, Rutka JA, Hawke M. The treatment of Ménière's disease: torok revisited. *Laryngoscope.* 1991;101:211–218.
8. Teufert KB, Berliner KI, De la Cruz A. Persistent dizziness after surgical treatment of vertigo: and exploratory study of prognostic factors. *Otol Neurotol.* 2007;28:1056–1062.
9. Thorp MA, Shehab ZP, Bance ML, Rutka JA. The AAO-HNS Committee on Hearing and Equilibrium guidelines for diagnosis and evaluation of therapy in Ménière's disease: have they been applied in the published literature of the last decade? *Clin Otolaryngol.* 2003;28:173–176.
10. Mikulec AA, Hartsock JJ, Salț AN. Permeability of the round window membrane is influenced by the composition of applied drug solutions and by common surgical procedures. *Otol Neurotol.* 2008;29(7):1020–1026.
11. Plontke SK, Biegner T, Kammerer B, Delabar U, Salt AN. Dexamethasone concentration gradients along scala tympani after application to the round

window membrane. *Otol Neurotol.* 2008; 29(3):401–406.
12. Ruckenstein MJ. Immunologic aspects of Ménière's disease. *Am J Otolaryngol.* 1999;20(3):161–165.
13. Parnes LS, Sun AH, Freeman DJ. Corticosteroid pharmacokinetics in the inner ear fluids: an animal study followed by clinical application. *Laryngoscope.* 1999; 109(7 pt 2):1–17.
14. Boleas-Aguirre MS, Lin FR, Della Santina CC, Minor LB, Carey JP. Longitudinal results with intratympanic dexamethasone in the treatment of Ménière's disease. *Otol Neurotol.* 2008;29(1):33–38.
15. Sennaroglu L, Sennaroglu G, Gursel B, Dini FM. Intratympanic dexamethasone, intratympanic gentamicin, and endolymphatic sac surgery for intractable vertigo in Ménière's disease. *Otolaryngol Head Neck Surg.* 2001;125:537–543.
16. Garduno-Anaya MA, Couthino De Toledo H, Hinojosa-Gonzalez R, et al. Dexamethasone inner ear perfusion by intratympanic injection in unilateral Ménière's disease: a two-year prospective, placebo-controlled, double-blind, randomized trial. *Otolaryngol Head Neck Surg.* 2005;133:285–294.
17. Silverstein H, Isaacson JE, Olds MJ, et al. Dexamethasone inner ear perfusion for the treatment of Ménière's disease: a prospective, randomized, double-blind, crossover trial. *Am J Otol.* 1998;19: 196–201.
18. Barrs DM. Intratympanic injections of dexamethasone for long-term control of vertigo. *Laryngoscope.* 2004;114(11): 1910–1914.
19. Rizzi MD, Hirose K. Aminoglycoside ototoxicity. *Curr Opin Otolaryngol Head Neck Surg.* 2007;15(5):352–357.
20. Schuknecht HF. Ablation therapy in the management of Ménière's disease. *Acta Otolaryngol.* 1957;132:1–42.
21. Beck C, Schmidt CL. 10 years of experience with intratympanically applied streptomycin (gentamicin) in the therapy of morbus Ménière. *Arch Otorhinolaryngol.* 1978;221:149–152.
22. Odkvist LM. Middle ear ototoxic treatment for inner ear disease. *Acta Otolaryngol (Stockh).* 1989;457(suppl):83–86.
23. Nedzelski JM, Bryce GE, Pfleiderer AG. Treatment of Ménière's disease with topical gentamicin: a preliminary report. *J Otolaryngol.* 1992;21:95–101.
24. Atlas J, Parnes S. Intratympanic gentamicin for intractable Ménière's disease: 5-year follow-up. *J Otolaryngol.* 2003;32: 288–293.
25. Harner SG, Driscoll CLW, Facer GW, Beatty CW, McDonald TJ. Long-term follow-up of transtympanic gentamicin for Ménière's syndrome. *Otol Neurotol.* 2001;22:210–214.
26. Bodmer D, Morong S, Alexander A, Chen JM, Nedzelski JM. Long-term control in patients after intratympanic gentamicin instillation for Ménière's disease. *Otol Neurotol.* 2007;28:1140–1144.
27. Schoendorf J, Neugebauer P, Michel O. Continuous intratympanic infusion of gentamicin through a microcatheter in Ménière's disease. *Otolaryngol Head Neck Surg.* 2001;124:203–207.
28. Nedzelski JM, Chiong CM, Fradet GF, Schessel DA, Bryce GE, Pfleiderer AG. Intratympanic gentamicin instillation as treatment for unilateral Ménière's disease: update of an ongoing study. *Am J Otol.* 1993;14:278–282.
29. Atlas J, Parnes S. Intratympanic gentamicin for intractable Ménière's disease: 5-year follow-up. *J Otolaryngol.* 2003;32: 288–293.
30. Hirsch BE, Kamerer DB. Intratympanic gentamicin therapy for Ménière's disease. *Am J Otol.* 1997;18:44–51.
31. Harner SG, Driscoll CLW, Facer GW, Beatty CW, McDonald TJ. Long-term follow-up of transtympanic gentamicin for Ménière's syndrome. *Otol Neurotol.* 2001;22:210–214.
32. Usami S, Abe S, Shinkawa H, Kimberling WJ. Sensorineural hearing loss

caused by mitochondrial DNA mutations: a special reference to the A1555G mutation. *J Commun Disord.* 1998;31:423–434.
33. Hu DN, Qui WQ, Wu BT, et al. Genetic aspects of antibiotic induced deafness: mitochondrial inheritance. *J Med Genet.* 1991;28:79–83.
34. Chen JM, Williamson PA, Hutchin T, Nedzelski JM, Cortopassi GA. Topical gentamicin-induced hearing loss: a mitochondrial ribosomal RNA study of genetic susceptibility. *Am J Otol.* 1996;17(6):850–852.
35. Salt AN, Gill RM, Plontke SK. Dependence of hearing changes on the dose of intratympanically applied gentamicin: a meta-analysis using mathematical simulations of clinical drug delivery protocols. *Laryngoscope.* 2008;118:1793–1800.
36. Chia SH, Garnst AC, Anderson JP, Harris JP. Intratympanic gentamicin therapy for Ménière's disease: a meta-analysis. *Otol Neurotol.* 2005;25:544–552.
37. Cohen-Kerem R, Kisilevsky V, Einarson TR, et al. Intratympanic Gentamicin for Ménière's disease: a meta-analysis. *Laryngoscope.* 2004;114:2085–2091.
38. Portmann G. Vertigo: surgical treatment by opening the saccus endolymphaticus. *Arch Otolaryngol.* 1927;6:309–319.
39. Smith WK, Sankar V, Pfleiderer AG. A national survey amongst UK otolaryngologists regarding the treatment of Ménière's disease. *J Laryngol Otol.* 2005;119:102–105.
40. Schuknecht HF. Myths in neurotology. *Am J Otol.* 1992;13:124–126.
41. Shambaugh GE, Clemis JD, Arenberg IK. Endolymphatic duct and sac in Ménière's disease. *Arch Otolaryngol.* 1969;89:816–825.
42. Gianoli CJ, LaRouere MJ, Kartush JM, et al. Sac-vein decompression for intractable Ménière's disease: two-year treatment results. *Otolaryngol Head Neck Surg.* 1998;188:22–29.
43. Graham MD, Kemink JL. Surgical management of Ménière's disease with endolymphatic sac decompression by wide bony decompression of the posterior fossa dura: technique and results. *Laryngoscope.* 1984;94:680–683.
44. House WF. Subarachnoid shunt for drainage of hydrops: a report of 63 cases. *Arch Otolaryngol.* 1964;79:338.
45. Brackmann DE, Nissen RL. Ménière's disease: results of treatment with the endolymphatic subarachnoid shunt compared with the endolymphatic mastoid shunt. *Am J Otolaryngol.* 1987;8:275–282.
46. Paparella MM, Sajjadi H. Endolymphatic sac enhancement. *Otolaryngol Clin North Am.* 1994;27:381–402.
47. Arenberg IK, Stahle J, Wilbrand H, Newkirk JB. Unidirectional inner ear valve implant for endolymphatic sac surgery in Ménière's disease. *Arch Otolaryngol.* 1978;104:694–704.
48. Jackson CG, Dickens JRE, Glasscock ME, et al. Endolymphatic system shunting: a long-term profile of the Denver Inner Ear Shunt. *Am J Otol.* 1996;17:85–88.
49. Telischi FF, Luxford WM. Long-term efficacy of endolymphatic sac surgery for vertigo in Ménière's disease. *Otolaryngol Head Neck Surg.* 1193;109:83–87.
50. Huang TS, Lin CC. Endolymphatic sac surgery for Ménière's disease: A composite study of 339 cases. *Laryngoscope.* 1985;95:1082–1086.
51. Moffat DA. Endolymphatic sac surgery: analysis of 100 operations. *Clin Otolaryngol.* 1994;19:261–266.
52. Huang TS, Lin CC. Endolymphatic sac ballooning surgery for Ménière's disease. *Ann Otol Rhinol Laryngol.* 1994;103:389–394.
53. Glasscock ME, Miller GW, Drake FD, Kanok MM. Surgical management of Ménière's disease with the endolymphatic subarachnoid shunt: A five-year study. *Laryngoscope.* 1977;87:1668–1675.
54. Brinson GM, Chen DA, Arriaga MA. Endolymphatic mastoid shunt versus endolymphatic sac decompression for

Ménière's disease. *Otolaryngol Head Neck Surg.* 2007;136:415–421.
55. Brackmann DE, Nissen RL. Ménière's Disease: results of treatment with the endolymphatic subarachnoid shunt compared with the endolymphatic mastoid shunt. *Am J Otol.* 1987;8:275–282.
56. Paparella MM, Hanson DG. Endolymphatic sac drainage for intractable vertigo (method and experiences). *Laryngoscope.* 1976;86:697–703.
57. Arenberg IK. The results of the first 300 consecutive endolymphatic system-mastoid shunts with valve implants for hydrops. *Otolaryngol Clin North Am.* 1983;16:153–168.
58. Arenberg IK. Results of endolymphatic sac to mastoid shunt surgery for Ménière's disease. *Am J Otol.* 1987;8:335–344.
59. Glasscock ME III. Current status on surgery for Ménière's disease. *Otolaryngol Head Neck Surg.* 1984;92:67–73.
60. Jackson CG, Dickens JRE, Glasscock ME, et al. Endolymphatic sac to mastoid shunt surgery using the Denver Inner Ear Shunt. *Otolaryngol Head Neck Surg.* 1988;99:282–285.
61. Morrison AM. Sac surgery on the only or better hearing ear. *Otolaryngol Clin North Am.* 1982;16:143–151.
62. Thomsen J, Bretlau P, Tos M, Johnsen NJ. Placebo effect in surgery for Ménière's Disease. *Arch Otolaryngol.* 1981;107:271–277.
63. Thomsen J, Bretlau P, Tos M, Johnsen NJ. Placebo effect in surgery for Ménière's disease: three-year follow up. *Otolaryngol Head Neck Surg.* 1983;91:183–186.
64. Thomsen J, Bretlau P, Tos M, Johnsen NJ. Endolymphatic sac-mastoid shunt surgery: a nonspecific treatment modality? *Ann Otol Rhinol Laryngol.* 1986;95:32–35.
65. Bretlau P, Thomsen J, Tos M, Johnsen NJ. Placebo effect in surgery for Ménière's disease: nine-year follow up. *Am J Otol.* 1989;10:259–261.
66. Pillsbury HC 3rd, Arenberg IK, Ferraro J, Ackley RS. Endolymphatic sac surgery. The Danish sham surgery study: an alternative analysis. *Otolaryngol Clin North Am.* 1983;16:123–127.
67. Welling DB, Nagaraja HN. Endolymphatic mastoid shunt: a reevaluation of efficacy. *Otolaryngol Head Neck Surg.* 2000;122:340–345.
68. Jackler RK, Whinney D. A century of eighth nerve surgery. *Otol Neurotol.* 2001;22:401–416.
69. Dandy WE. Ménière's disease: its diagnosis and a method of treatment. *Arch Surg.* 1928;16:1127–1152.
70. House WF. Surgical exposure of the internal auditory canal and its contents through the middle cranial fossa. *Laryngoscope.* 1961;71:1363–1385.
71. Fisch U. Vestibular nerve section for Ménière's disease. *Am J Otol.* 1984;5:543–545.
72. Glasscock ME, Johnson GD, Poe DE. Long-term hearing results following middle fossa vestibular nerve section. *Otolaryngol Head Neck Surg.* 1989;100:35–40.
73. Smyth GD, Kerr AG, Primrose W. Operations on the saccus endolymphaticus and vestibular nerve: have they fulfilled their promise? *Otolaryngol Head Neck Surg.* 1986;94:594–600.
74. Garcia-Ibanez E, Garcia-Ibanez JL. Middle fossa vestibular neurectomy: a report of 373 cases. *Otolaryngol Head Neck Surg.* 1980;88:486–490.
75. Gavilan J, Gavilan C. Middle fossa vestibular neurectomy; long term results. *Arch Otolaryngol.* 1984;110:785–787.
76. Silverstein H, Norrell H. Retrolabyrinthine surgery: a direct approach to the cerebellopontine angle. *Otolaryngol Head Neck Surg.* 1980;88:462–469.
77. Silverstein H, Norrell H, Haberkamp T. A comparison of retrosigmoid IAC, retrolabyrinthine, and middle fossa vestibular neurectomy for treatment of vertigo. *Laryngoscope.* 1987;97:165–173.
78. Glasscock ME 3rd, Thedinger BA, Cueva RA, Jackson CG. An analysis of the retrolabyrinthine vs. the retrosigmoid

vestibular nerve section. *Otolaryngol Head Neck Surg.* 1991;104:88–95.

79. Nguyen CD, Brackmann DE, Crane RT, Linthicum FH Jr, Hitselberger WE. Retrolabyrinthine vestibular nerve section: evaluation of technical modification in 143 cases. *Am J Otol.* 1992;13:328–332.
80. Glasscock ME 3rd, Thedinger BA, Cueva RA, Jackson CG. An analysis of the retrolabyrinthine vs. the retrosigmoid vestibular nerve section. *Otolaryngol Head Neck Surg.* 1991;104(1):88–95.
81. Fukuhara T, Silverman DA, Hughes GB, et al. Vestibular nerve sectioning for intractable vertigo: efficacy of simplified retrosigmoid approach. *Otol Neurotol.* 2002:23(1):67–72.
82. Kaylie DM, Jackson CG, Gardner EK. Surgical management of Ménière's disease in the era of gentamicin. *Otolaryngol Head Neck Surg.* 2005;132(3):443–450.
83. Silverstein H, Norrell H, Smouha EE. Retrosigmoid-internal auditory canal approach vs. retrolabyrinthine approach for vestibular neurectomy. *Otolaryngol Head Neck Surg.* 1987;97:300–307.
84. McKenna MJ, Nadol JB Jr, Ojemann RG, Halpin C. Vestibular neurectomy: retrosigmoid-intracanalicular versus retrolabyrinthine approach. *Am J Otol.* 1996;17:253–258.
85. Berryhill WE, Graham MD. Chemical and physical labyrinthectomy for Ménière's disease. *Otolaryngol Clin North Am.* 2002;35(3):675–682.
86. Colletti V, Fiorino FG, Sittoni V. NaCl deposition in the vestibule: a simple, safe, and effective method of cochleovestibular deafferentiation. *Am J Otol.* 1989;10:451–455.
87. Stahle J. Ultrasonic treatment of Ménière's disease. *Acta Otolaryngol (Stockh).* 1988;106(suppl 449):11–12.
88. Wolfson RJ. Labyrinthine cryosurgery for Ménière's disease:present status. *Otolaryngol Head Neck Surg.* 1984;92: 221–224.
89. Linthicum FH Jr, Alonso A, Denia A. Traumatic neuroma: a complication of transcanal labyrinthectomy. *Arch Otolaryngol.* 1979;105:654–655.
90. Langman AW, Lindeman RC. Surgery for vertigo in the nonserviceable hearing ear: transmastoid labyrinthectomy or translabyrinthine vestibular nerve section. *Laryngoscope.* 1993;103:1321–1325.
91. De La Cruz A, Teufert KB, Berliner KI. Transmastoid labyrinthectomy versus translabyrinthine vestibular nerve section: does cutting the vestibular nerve make a difference in outcome? *Otol Neurotol.* 2007;28:801–808.
92. Lustig L, Yeagle J, Niparko JK, Minor LB. Cochlear implantation in patients with bilateral Ménière's syndrome. *Otol Neurotol.* 2003;24:397–403.

12

Rehabilitation of the Patient With Ménière's Disease

Elizabeth Grace, PT, MS, NCS

Introduction

People with Ménière's disease often have symptoms of vertigo, dizziness, imbalance, or combinations of these. The course of the disease varies greatly and affects people differently. Vestibular rehabilitation physical therapy can make a significant functional impact on a patient's ability to perform routine daily activities and on his or her quality of life.

Traditionally, vestibular rehabilitation has not been utilized extensively with patients with Ménière's because the disease is often considered an unstable, fluctuating vestibular lesion not amenable to vestibular therapy. However, over the past 20 years, a great deal of literature has been published demonstrating and discussing the appropriateness of vestibular rehabilitation in patients' with Ménière's disease. There are many times throughout the course of the disease when a patient may benefit from participation in a vestibular rehabilitation program. It has been suggested by various sources that delaying vestibular rehabilitation can lead to chronic symptoms and poor compensatory habits, which may be difficult to reverse. Even more unfortunate is the situation where conservative treatment is not considered before invasive and permanent procedures are performed, when the patient's complaints and functional limitations may have been resolved with a simple course of rehabilitation.

This chapter reviews what vestibular rehabilitation is, when it is not appropriate, and more importantly, discusses the various indications for this form of therapy. Additionally, case studies are presented to illustrate the various uses of vestibular rehabilitation for patients with Ménière's disease.

What Is Vestibular Rehabilitation?

Vestibular rehabilitation, also called balance rehabilitation, or vestibular and balance rehabilitation therapy (VBRT), is a noninvasive, exercise-based treatment approach to facilitating central nervous system processes to produce compensatory responses for the patient with dizziness and/or imbalance. Vestibular rehabilitation uses existing neural mechanisms in the brain for adaptation, plasticity, and compensation.

Goals of VBRT include:

- Decrease or eliminate dizziness/vertigo
- Improve gaze stabilization and visual motor control
- Improve tolerance to motion—self-motion and motion in the environment
- Improve functional balance and safety
- Educate the patient in safety and compensation strategies to control their symptoms
- Increase activity levels
- Reduce falls or risks for falls
- Decrease associated symptoms
- Increase functional independence at home, work, and in the community
- Educate the patient regarding the nature of the disease process, the role that rehabilitation can play in decreasing functional deficits and limitations and the expected course and goals of a rehabilitation program.

The use of exercises to treat patients with dizziness was first introduced in the 1940s by the otolaryngologist Sir Terence Cawthorne and the physiotherapist F. S. Cooksey. Cawthorne-Cooksey exercises are a generic program of a variety of eye, head, and body movements to habituate to dizziness. More recent studies, however, demonstrate that customized VBRT programs are more effective than generic exercise programs.[1–3] Progress in understanding the complexity of vestibular disorders has enabled vestibular specialists to prescribe treatment interventions that are more specific to different disease processes. Additionally, this more customized approach allows the therapy program to be tailored to the individual needs of each patient, which is preferred, as patients with Ménière's disease present with such varied complaints and functional difficulties. Based on the findings from a thorough evaluation, an appropriate therapy program can be designed to address the specific deficits, needs, and circumstances of each patient.

For best results, patients should be referred to therapists with specialized training in vestibular rehabilitation. Inappropriate treatment by an unskilled therapist can make a patient feel significantly worse, which may delay appropriate care or may prevent a patient from continuing with a therapy program.[4–6] Therapists considered vestibular specialists will have participated in postgraduate education courses on vestibular dysfunction and rehabilitation that present evidence-based concepts of vestibular dysfunction and recovery and practical application of those concepts.

A thorough vestibular examination includes vestibular system-specific tests to identify the type of vestibular deficit (unilateral, bilateral, central, multifactorial balance deficit), and assessment of functional limitations and deficits. Use of standardized and validated outcome measures should also be included in the assessment. These may include, but are not limited to, the Dynamic Gait Index (DGI),[7] Functional Gait Assessment (FGA),[8] Dizziness Handicap Inventory (DHI),[9] Activities-Specific Balance Confidence scale (ABC),[10] and Disability Scale.[11]

Interventions utilized in vestibular and balance rehabilitation include gaze stabilization exercises (adaptation and substitution exercises), sensory integration activities, habituation exercises (for self-motion and also visual motion in the environment), postural control exercises (both static and dynamic balance activities), and encouragement of increased activity levels via guarded practice in a safe environment and guided progression of activity in home program. The therapist can get very creative in ways to work on deficit areas with a fun and functional approach.

When Is Vestibular and Balance Rehabilitation *NOT* Indicated?

Vestibular and balance rehabilitation has many indications and benefits. However, it is not indicated for the patient who experiences *only* spontaneous episodes of true vertigo, with no precipitating cause or activity. In between these episodes, patients have normal balance and vestibular function. This would be considered a fluctuating, unstable lesion and would not generally respond to vestibular rehabilitation.[1,12–14] Additionally, if patients experience frequent spontaneous episodes of vertigo, this also indicates the lesion is unstable and the patient may not be appropriate for vestibular rehabilitation. Once the frequency of episodes is controlled, the patient may then be appropriate for a referral to therapy.

When *Is* Vestibular and Balance Rehabilitation Indicated?

There are many indications for VBRT for patients with Ménière's disease. The efficacy of this type of modality has been studied extensively and shown to be beneficial in many circumstances. These include:

- New diagnosis education (or education at a later stage of disease)
- Benign paroxysmal positional vertigo
- Uncompensated vestibular lesions from progressive labyrinthine dysfunction
- Bilateral vestibular loss (bilateral Ménière's disease)
- Pre and/or postgentamicin injection therapy
- Pre/postablative surgery
- General functional balance disorders.

New Diagnosis Patient Education

A diagnosis of Ménière's disease can be overwhelming for many patients. Educating patients on various topics related to their disease is essential in facilitating patients' understanding of their disease and their ability to become self-empowered to take control of an unpredictable disease. Therapists are typically allotted more one on one time with patients, compared with physicians, which can adjunct the physicians' education of patients on various topics. In this age of technology, patients often will search the Internet to find additional information about their disease. This can be a useful resource, however, it can also lead to patients finding inaccurate information or information not applicable to their individual situation. Rehabilitation specialists can play a key role in reviewing this information with the patient and can best guide them to appropriate resources.

The idea of employing vestibular rehabilitation to encourage education, prevention, and self-empowerment, suggested by Dowdal-Osborn in 2002,[14] is a different line of thinking than the traditionally accepted notion of referring patients to vestibular rehabilitation only for decreasing symptoms through specific exercises aimed at adaptation, habituation, and postural control retraining. Whitney and Rossi (2000)[4] suggested that vestibular rehabilitation is appropriate for newly diagnosed patients during an inactive phase of the disease to educate patients on the disease process and various resources available, such as support groups. Furthermore, patients should be educated on fall prevention during a Ménière's attack of vertigo.

Benign Paroxysmal Positional Vertigo—BPPV

BPPV is one of the most common causes of dizziness. Patients with Ménière's disease are predisposed to this common disorder. Various authors have looked at this population of patients with Ménière's disease and BPPV.[15–18] Gananca et al[15] found that patients with Ménière's disease and BPPV had nystagmus and vertigo eliminated with 1, 2, or 3 Epley maneuvers. Conversely, Gross et al[17] found that Ménière's disease may predispose patients to intractable BPPV. Nevertheless, given the enormous amount of literature demonstrating the effectiveness of treatment for BPPV,[19–22] patients with Ménière's disease who are also found to have BPPV should be treated for this disorder. Vestibular rehabilitation also may be indicated for patients with motion sensitivity following BPPV, when the BPPV itself is no longer active, but the patient continues to experience movement sensitivity.

Peripheral Vestibular Damage

Progressive Uncompensated Vestibular Hypofunction

Over time, many patients with Ménière's disease will experience a progressive loss of vestibular function and will present with signs and symptoms of unilateral vestibular hypofunction. There is no clearly identified rule regarding how infrequent spontaneous events should be for vestibular rehabilitation to be recommended and successful.[12] If a patient appears relatively stable, with occasional spontaneous, unprovoked episodes of vertigo, yet additionally reports symptoms consistent with unilateral hypofunction between these spontaneous events, vestibular rehabilitation should be considered.[1,12,23]

Shepard and Telian[1] suggested vestibular rehabilitation can be utilized to help determine if a patient's complaints are the result of unstable labyrinthine function or an uncompensated vestibular loss. If a course of therapy decreases the patient's complaints, more aggressive treatment can be avoided. However, if symptoms are not controlled through therapy, ablative or surgical procedures may need to be considered. A trial of this noninvasive treatment may be beneficial prior to resorting to procedures that will cause permanent damage.

In 2005, Gottshall et al[24] demonstrated efficacy of vestibular rehabilitation on symptoms of unsteadiness and dysequilibrium, once episodic vertigo had been controlled with medical therapy alone. Prior to this study, little work had demonstrated the use of vestibular rehabilitation in patients with Ménière's disease, except following ablative and surgical procedures. Patients in this study were treated with diuretic therapy or transtympanic steroid injections for episodic vertigo. Once patients were vertigo-free for 3 months, they started vestibular rehabilitation. Eighty-eight percent of patients reported resolution of pretreatment unsteadiness. Patients also made improvements in scores for computerized posturography, Dizziness Handicap Inventory, Dynamic Gait Index, and Activities-Specific Balance Confidence scale. The results of this study support the use of vestibular rehabilitation in patients with Ménière's disease.

Bilateral Vestibular Hypofunction

Approximately one-third of patients with Ménière's disease have bilateral involvement, which may lead to bilateral vestibular hypofunction.[23,25] As with patients with bilateral vestibular loss from other causes, patients often have little remaining vestibular function, and therefore the focus of vestibular rehabilitation is on helping patients substitute for that loss, using alternative strategies, while enhancing the use of any remaining vestibular function. Extensive patient education and reduction of fall risk are important aspects of rehabilitation for these patients. Although, prognosis is more guarded for patients with bilateral hypofunction than for those with unilateral involvement, vestibular rehabilitation is appropriate and effective.[1,4,12,26–28]

Pre- and/or Postgentamicin Injection Therapy

When a patient's episodes of vertigo are not controlled with diet or medical therapy, ablative procedures may be considered.[6,29–33] The purpose of ablative procedures, such as intratympanic gentamicin injections, is to control vertigo by partially or completely destroying the vestibular labyrinth, while preserving hearing. This procedure will change an unstable, fluctuating lesion into a stable lesion that often will respond to traditional vestibular rehabilitation techniques for treating vestibular hypofunction.

Several researchers report on unsteadiness and decreased postural control resulting from gentamicin injections[6,29,31]; yet physicians often delay referrals to vestibular rehabilitation, believing the deficits will go away with time. However, earlier referrals to therapy may result in patients' experiencing less functional deficits and quicker return to full functional activity levels.

In many patients, only a few treatment sessions, along with a home-based program, are needed to achieve significant or full resolution of symptoms. If the physician has concerns that a patient may have more difficulty with loss of vestibular function following ablation, the patient can be referred to vestibular rehabilitation prior to the start of the gentamicin treatment. This will start the process of compensation and thorough education before the patient has the loss of function. Although vestibular rehabilitation is recommended frequently in the literature on intratympanic gentamicin use in Ménière's disease,[6,31–34] this modality may not be used as frequently as is indicated by patients' complaints and needs further investigation to demonstrate its efficacy.

Pre- and/or Postablative Surgical Procedures

Ablative surgical procedures (labyrinthectomy and vestibular nerve section), although sometimes necessary to eliminate vertigo, leave patients with an acute unilateral loss of vestibular function. Vestibular rehabilitation is an essential compliment to any ablative surgical procedure to assist patients' return to full function without symptoms.[4,12,35] In some cases, it is helpful for patients to be seen by a vestibular specialist prior to surgery to instruct the patient on adaptation exercises that will be started shortly after surgery. When patients are familiar with the exercises, it is much easier for them to start performing them following surgery, rather than trying to learn new exercises when they are just recovering from the surgery.

Patients should ideally be seen in the acute care setting following surgery by a therapist with knowledge of vestibular rehabilitation to get started with a walking program and vestibular adaptation exercises prior to leaving the hospital. If possible, patients should then be referred to an outpatient vestibular therapist. In all likelihood, patients will naturally compensate following ablative surgery; however, vestibular rehabilitation can facilitate complete compensation and recovery of full function without symptoms in a more timely manner. The symptoms and functional limitations that patients report following ablative surgeries can be quite disruptive to normal functioning and the impact therapy can make on a patient's life can be quite significant. For example, being able to return to work at a fully functional level or being able to complete all household chores without evoking symptoms just 1 to 2 weeks sooner can make significant difference in a patient's life. Again, the therapy program often requires just a few treatment sessions with a mainly home-based program.

Research has demonstrated the benefits of vestibular rehabilitation following vestibular surgeries.[4,12,35–37] Mruzek et al[35] found patients had less motion sensitivity and dizziness handicap following vestibular rehabilitation after ablation surgeries, indicating more rapid and complete recovery. Patients following ablation surgeries present similarly to those postacoustic neuroma resection. El Kashlan et al[37] found 68% of patients following surgery for acoustic neuroma resections were able to walk independently 1 week after surgery and 89% of patients who had vestibular rehabilitation felt it had improved their condition. Herdman et al[36] found patients who had vestibular therapy in the acute-care hospital following acoustic neuroma resections had a decreased sense of dysequilibrium and improved postural stability.

General Functional Balance Disorders

Vestibular and balance rehabilitation therapy can and should also be utilized when a patient has any functional balance disorder. This disorder may be a direct result of vestibular dysfunction or may be a multifactorial functional problem. Nonetheless, a thorough rehabilitation program can assess what may be causing the functional problems and address all areas needing improvement. Another important aspect of any balance assessment is a falls-risk evaluation and remediation of problem areas. Patient/family education is often a key component of this intervention.

Case Illustrations

Case Study 1—PK

PK is a 54-year-old female diagnosed with Ménière's disease 2 years ago, after a 6-year history of vertigo and dizziness. She had 3 gentamicin injections last year and underwent a successful course of vestibular rehabilitation after the injections, after which she reported no symptoms or functional complaints.

Patient presents to therapy with 3-month history of significant imbalance, general movement sensitivity, and sensitivity to visual motion in her environment. Symptoms are episodic and occur every 1 to 2 weeks. PK also has more constant symptoms of imbalance with any walking, especially outdoors. Symptoms are rated as 5/10 on average, 6 to 7/10 at worst. Additionally, she reports 2 falls in the past 3 months, each occurring while walking outside.

Past medical history other than Ménière's disease is significant for HTN, hyperlipidemia, and breast cancer 9 years ago with associated lymphedema. Patient lives with her adult disabled daughter and works part-time as a crossing guard. She reports that she sometimes does get symptoms while working and is particularly stimulated by the cars passing by her corner. She has not informed her employer about her Ménière's disease and is very concerned that she will lose her job because of her functional difficulties. She does not use any assistive devices or other equipment.

Clinical examination reveals normal oculomotor testing, normal head thrust test, normal vestibular testing with fixation removed, and normal reactive and anticipatory balance reactions. On the Modified Clinical Test of Sensory Interaction on Balance (mCTSIB), patient was able to hold 4 of 4 test positions for 30 sec, with increased difficulty with eyes closed on firm surface and significant difficulty with eyes closed on foam. Patient also had significant difficulty with tandem stance and single leg stance, especially with eyes closed. Dynamic Gait Index score was 17/24, indicating patient is at increased risk for falling. The most difficult activities for the patient were walking while making head turns, stepping over an object, and stair climbing. Patient ambulates without assistive device with slightly widened base of support and decreased gait speed, based on age-related norms. Dizziness Handicap Inventory score is 52/100. Activity-Specific Balance Confidence score is 77%. Disability scale is rated as 3—symptoms currently disrupt social and exercise activities and to a mild extent disrupt my work.

PK attended 6 sessions of therapy over 9 weeks. Due to her schedule, she was unable to attend more frequent sessions, however did report daily compliance to her home exercise program. Her in-therapy and home exercise program consisted of various static and dynamic balance exercises, a walking program performed in a busy environment, optokinetic stimulation training to decrease visual motion sensitivity, and extensive patient education.

At discharge, her Dynamic Gait Index score is 20/24; Dizziness Handicap Inventory score is 18/100; Activities-specific Balance Confidence scale score is 88%; and Disability score is 2. She is able to hold 4 of 4 positions on the modified clinical test of sensory interaction on balance (mCTSIB) without significant difficulty and has less difficulty maintaining tandem stance and single leg stance with eyes open and eyes closed. She rates her symptom intensity as 2 to 3/10 at worst and 0.5/10 on average. She is able to work and perform daily household activities, including caring for her daughter, without significant difficulty.

Case Study 2—MW

MW is a 48-year-old male who was diagnosed with Ménière's disease 2 years ago. He received his first gentamicin injection 2 weeks ago. He reports experiencing an episode of true vertigo approximately 1 week later. He presents to therapy at this time with chief complaint of feeling "woozy" and significantly off balance, with difficulty ambulating. Additionally, he reports symptoms associated with head movement and position changes. In the past week, he rates his symptoms on a 0 to 10 scale as 5/10 at best and 9/10 at worst.

Past medical history is insignificant, other than the Ménière's disease. He lives with his family, including 3 young children and works full-time as a sales manager. He currently is independent with ADLs, but is having difficulty performing normal household duties. He also is normally very physically active, including golf, swimming, and other outdoor activities. Currently, he is not performing any of these activities.

Clinical examination is significant for normal oculomotor exam, normal gaze-evoked nystagmus (without fixation), positive Post Head-Shake test for right beating nystagmus, and positive left Head Thrust test. On the mCTSIB, he was able to hold 3/4 positions for 30 sec. He had difficulty with eyes closed on firm surface and was only able to hold stance on foam surface with eyes closed for 3 sec. Gait assessment is unremarkable, with the exception of mild imbalance noted. Dynamic Gait Index score is 20/24, with difficulty noted with head turns, stepping over objects, and he required use of a railing on stairs. His Dizziness Handicap Inventory score is 48/100. Disability scale is 3. Activity-Specific Balance Confidence scale score is 66%.

During MW's initial session, he was instructed on a daily walking program, balance exercises, and gaze stability exercises for compensation of vestibular dysfunction. Over the course of his rehabilitation, these exercises were progressed and more challenging exercises were added to his program. He performed mostly a home-based program and, in total, attended 3 therapy sessions over 7 weeks.

At discharge, MW's Dynamic Gait Index score is 24/24. He is able to maintain 4/4 positions on the mCTSIB for

30 sec without difficulty. Dizziness Handicap Inventory score is 4/100. Disability score is 0. Activities-Specific Balance Confidence score is 97%. He rated his symptoms as 0/10. He reports he had returned to all normal daily functional activities and recreational activities, as prior to the gentamicin injections.

Case Study 3—DS

DS is a 58-year-old female diagnosed with Ménière's disease 10 years ago, which has worsened over time. More recently, she reports a new onset of dizziness beginning approximately 1 year ago, which resolved within two months; however returned about 8 months ago. She reports the symptoms have worsened over the past 2 weeks, with more position-change related vertigo, which is different from her other symptoms. In addition to this positional vertigo, she reports she is generally off-balance and has general movement sensitivity. She rated her position-provoked symptoms as 8 of 10 on a 0 to 10 scale and her imbalance as 5 of 10.

Other than the Ménière's disease, her past medical history is significant for hypertension. She lives with her husband and elderly father. She works full-time for a billing department of a community hospital. She is independent with ADLs; however, reports these activities are difficult for her. Currently, she is not working and is not performing her normal household chores, yard work, or social/recreational activities.

She was involved in a motor vehicle accident 3 weeks ago, where she drove into a tree on her neighbor's front lawn after experiencing an episode of vertigo while driving. She has a chest contusion and some additional bruises from this recent MVA. She was evaluated at a local emergency department and found to not have any more significant injuries.

DS had a complete vestibular function test performed three months prior to the referral to therapy. At that time, she reported episodic subjective vertigo lasting minutes to hours, occurring daily. Testing demonstrated a significant left vestibular hypofunction without significant additional findings. Her Sensory Organization test was within normal limits.

Clinical examination is significant for normal oculomotor exam, gaze evoked nystagmus (without fixation), and post-head-shake nystagmus. Left Head Thrust test is positive. Gait assessment is significant for a slow, cautious gait, which patient reports has been her pattern since her MVA due to pain and discomfort. She also is slow and cautious with bed mobility and functional transfers. Dynamic Gait Index deferred at initial assessment. Dizziness Handicap Inventory score is 72/100.

Additionally, Dix-Hallpike testing was positive for left torsional, upbeating nystagmus, lasting 15 sec, associated with subjective report of vertigo. This finding is indicative of benign paroxysmal positional vertigo of the left posterior canal. DS was treated during this session with a left canalith repositioning maneuver (CRT), performed twice.

She returned the following week with no significant improvement in complaints. She reported 3 episodes of true vertigo, each lasting approximately 1 minute. Each episode occurred following head or body movement. She also reported feeling "off-balance" 90%

of the time. Upon Dix-Hallpike testing, left torsional, upbeating nystagmus was again noted, however, with less intensity and shorter duration (approximately 6 sec). Patient was again treated with left CRT × 2. Upon second CRT, no symptoms or nystagmus was noted in the Dix-Hallpike position of the CRT treatment.

At the next treatment the following week, patient reported decreased positional nystagmus; however, she continued to experience episodes of subjective vertigo, lasting approximately 1 minute each. Dix-Hallpike testing was negative for nystamgus, with mild symptoms noted on testing of both left and right sides. Vestibular compensation exercises and balance exercises were initiated and added to a home exercise program. DS attended 4 additional sessions of therapy, at which her program was progressed as appropriate and tolerated. Considerable patient education was included in her therapy program, including topics on the nature of her disorder, the role of rehabilitation, expected course of care and goals of therapy, effect of anxiety on symptoms of dizziness and additional treatments available.

DS continued to report spontaneous episodes of vertigo, each lasting 1 to 2 minutes. Although she continued to make functional improvements and improved on objective measures of function and balance, she continued to express significant concern with being able to return to her normal daily activities. She appeared to have significant anxiety associated with return of her symptoms and she was very fearful of having another severe incident, such as her motor vehicle accident. After consulting with her referring otorhinolaryngologist, he assessed her comorbidity of anxiety and the effect on her complaints of dizziness and started her on Effexor. She responded very well to the combination of vestibular rehabilitation and medication.

In total, she attended 8 sessions of therapy over 16 weeks. At discharge, her Dynamic Gait Index score was 23/24; Dizziness Handicap Inventory score was 6/100; and Disability score was 1. She was able to maintain 3/4 positions on the mCTSIB without significant difficulty. She was unable to maintain balance on foam surface with her eyes closed for >15 sec. She was able to maintain balance with tandem and single leg stance with eyes open for 30 seconds; however had difficulty maintaining these positions with her eyes closed. She rated her symptoms as 0/10. She reported that she had returned to all previous activities, including work, driving, household activities, and social activities. She did note experiencing occasional (2 to 3 × per week) brief episodes of dizziness, lasting only seconds, which occurred with quick head movements. These symptoms were not of significant concern to her. Her home exercise program was progressed and patient education was completed at that final session.

Summary

The effects of Ménière's disease on a person's quality of life and functional abilities can be quite severe. Vestibular rehabilitation offers a noninvasive treatment option to address and improve many impairments facing people with Ménière's disease, at various stages of the disease. This treatment option may successfully address the functional complaints of patients with Ménière's disease, preventing or delaying the need for permanent, more invasive procedures.

An experienced vestibular rehabilitation specialist works with individuals to problem-solve issues and difficulties, and design and progress individualized exercise programs appropriate to individual needs to promote safety and functional independence. The proper implementation of specialized vestibular treatment has been shown to greatly improve the person's overall quality of life. Further work is needed to demonstrate the efficacy of vestibular rehabilitation at various stages of the disease process; yet given the demonstrated benefits of vestibular rehabilitation for patients with Ménière's disease, its use should be considered when determining the best treatment plan for complaints associated with Ménière's disease.

References

1. Shepard NT, Telian SA. Programmatic vestibular rehabilitation. *Otolaryngol Head Neck Surg.* 1995;112(1):173–182.
2. Shepard NT, Telian SA, Smith-Wheelock M, Raj A. Vestibular and balance rehabilitation therapy. *Ann Otol Rhinol Laryngol.* 1993;102:198–204.
3. Shumway-Cook A, Horak FB. Rehabilitation strategies for patients with vestibular deficits. *Neurol Clin.* 1990;8: 441–457.
4. Whitney SL, Metzinger Rossi M. Efficacy of vestibular rehabilitation. *Otolaryngol Clin North Am.* 2000;33:659–672.
5. Sajjadi H. Medical management of Ménière's disease. *Otolaryngol Clin North Am.* 2002;35:581–589.
6. Assimakopoulos D, Patrikakos G. Treatment of Ménière's disease by intratympanic gentamicin application. *J Laryngol Otol.* 2003;117:10–16.
7. Shumway-Cook A, Woollacott MH. *Motor Control: Theory and Practical Applications.* Baltimore, MD: Williams and Wilkins; 1995.
8. Wrisley DM, Marchetti GF, Kuharsky DK, Whitney SL. Reliability, internal consistency and validity of data obtained with the functional gait assessment. *Phys Ther.* 2004;84(10):906–918.
9. Jacobson GP, Newman CW. The development of the Dizziness Handicap Inventory. *Arch Otolaryngol Head Neck Surg.* 1990;116(4):424–427.
10. Powell LE, Myers AM. The activities-specific balance confidence (ABC) scale. *J Gerontol A Biol Sci Med Sci.* 1995; 50A(1):M28–34.
11. Shepard NT, Telian SA, Smith-Wheelock M. Habituation and balance retraining. A retrospective review. *Neurol Clin.* 1990;8(2):459–475.
12. Clendaniel RA, Tucci DL. Vestibular rehabilitation strategies in Ménière's disease. *Otolaryngol Clin North Am.* 1997;30:1145–1159.
13. Sajjadi H, Paparella MM. Ménière's disease. *Lancet.* 2008;372:406–414.
14. Dowdal-Osborn, M. *Otolaryngol Clin North Am.* 2002;35:683–690.
15. Gananca CF, Caovilla HH, Gazzola JM, et al. Epley's maneuver in benign paroxysmal positional vertigo associated with Ménière's disease. *Rev Bras Otorrinolaringol.* 2007;73(4):506–512.
16. Handa PR, Kuhn AMB, Cunha F, et al. Quality of life in patients with benign paroxysmal postional vertigo and/or Ménière's disease. *Rev Bras Otorrinolaringol.* 2005;71(6):776–783.
17. Gross EM, Ress BD, Viirre ES, Nelson JR, Harris JP. Intractable benign paroxysmal positional vertigo in patients with Ménière's disease. *Laryngoscope.* 2000;110:655–659.
18. Perez N, Martin E, Zubieta JL, et al. Benign paroxysmal positional vertigo in patients with Ménière's disease treated with intratympanic gentamycin. *Laryngoscope.* 2002;112:1104–1109.

19. Bhattacharyya N, Baugh RF, Orvidas L, et al. Clinical practice guideline: benign paroxysmal positional vertigo. *Otolaryngol Head Neck Surg.* 2008;139(5 suppl 4): S47–S81.
20. Teixeira LJ, Machado JN. Maneuvers for the treatment of benign positional paroxysmal vertigo: a systematic review. *Braz J Otorhinolaryngol.* 2006;72(1): 130–139.
21. Hilton M, Pinder D. The Epley ("canalith repositioning" manoeuvre for benign paroxysmal positional vertigo. *Cocharane Database Syst Rev.* 2004;2:CD003162.
22. Fife, TD, Lverson DJ, Lempert T, et al. Practice parameter: therapies for benign paroxysmal positional vertigo (an evidence-based review): report of the Quality Standards Subcommittee of the American Academy of Neurology. *Neurology.* 2008;70(22):2067–2074.
23. Hallpike C, Cairns H. Observations on the pathology of Ménière's syndrome. *J Laryngol.* 1938;53:625.
24. Gottshall KR, Hoffer ME, Moore RJ, Balough BJ. The role of vestibular rehabilitation in the treatment of Ménière's disease. *Otolaryngol Head Neck Surg.* 2005;133(3):326–238.
25. Wladislavosky-Waserman P, Farcer GQ, Mokri B, et al. Ménière's disease: a 30 year epidemiologic and clinical study in Rochester MN, 1951–1980. *Laryngoscope.* 1984;94:1098.
26. Telian SA, Shepard NT, Smith-Wheelock M, Hoberg M. Bilateral vestibular paresis: diagnosis and treatment. *Otolaryngol Head Neck Surg.* 1991;104:67–71.
27. Krebs DE, Gill-Body KM, Riley PO, Parker SW. Double-blind, placebo-controlled trial of rehabilitation for bilateral vestibular hypofunction; preliminary report. *Otolarynogol Head Neck Surg.* 1993;109: 735–741.
28. Whitney SL, Borello-France D. Bilateral vestibular disease: an overview. *Neurol Rep.* 1996;20:41–45.
29. Carey J. Intratympanic gentamicin for the treatment of Ménière's disease and other forms of peripheral vertigo. *Otolaryngol Clin North Am.* 2004;37:1075–1090.
30. Cohen-Karem R, Kisilevsky V, Einarson TR, et al. Intratympanic gentamicin for Ménière's disease: a meta-analysis. *Laryngoscope.* 2004;114:2085–2091.
31. Boleas-Aguirre MS, Sanchez-Ferrandiz N, Guillen-Grima F, Perez N. Long-term disability of class a patients with Ménière's disease after treatment with intratympanic gentamicin. *Laryngoscope.* 2007;117:1474–1481.
32. Suryanarayanan R, Cook JA. Long-term results of gentamicin inner ear perfusion in Ménière's disease. *J Laryngol Otol.* 2004;117:489–495.
33. Odkvist LM, Bergenius J, Moller C. When and how to use gentamicin in the treatment of Ménière's disease. *Acta Otolaryngol Suppl.* 1997;526:54–57.
34. Odkvist L. Gentamicin cures vertigo, but what happens to hearing? *Int Tinnitus J.* 1997;3(2):133–136.
35. Mruzek M, Barin K, Nichols DS, Burnett CN, Welling DB. Effects of vestibular rehabilitation and social reinforcement on recovery following ablative vestibular surgery. *Laryngoscope.* 1995;105: 686–692.
36. Herdman SJ, Clendaniel RA, Mattox DE, et al. Vestibular adaptation exercises and recovery: acute stage after acoustic neuroma resection. *Otolarynogol Head Neck Surg.* 1995;13:77–86.
37. El-Kashlan HK, Shepard NT, Arts A, et al. Disability from vestibular symptoms after acoustic neuroma resection. *Am J Otol.* 1998;19:104–111.

13

Psychological Attributes of Ménière's Disease

Jeffrey P. Staab, MD, MS

Introduction

Reports about suspected psychological causes or consequences of Ménière's disease date back more than 60 years. Early papers offered psychoanalytic formulations of this condition.[1] Later work investigated the possibility that psychosocial stress might trigger the onset of Ménière's disease or promote recurrent attacks.[2–4] Recent investigations examined the prevalence of anxiety and depressive disorders in patients with active and quiescent Ménière's disease[5–9] and the relationship between personality traits and susceptibility to Ménière's.[10–12] There are no controlled trials of treatment for psychological symptoms in patients with Ménière's disease, although subjects with Ménière's have been included in open label studies of antidepressants for patients with chronic dizziness.[13–15] This chapter examines the work of investigators from several disciplines who have attempted to shed light on the psychological attributes of patients with Ménière's disease, the role of stress in disease progression, and positive and negative behavioral changes experienced by individuals with Ménière's disease. As with all scientific endeavors, these investigations are products of their times, starting with the heyday of psychoanalytic theory in 1950s, advancing through stress-disease models of the 1960s and structured psychiatric classification systems of the 1980s, and culminating with recent interest in temperament and gene-environment interactions. Special attention is paid to observations made repeatedly across time, regardless of the theoretical bent of investigators, as these may hold the greatest value.

Stress, Personality Traits, and Ménière's Disease

The largest percentage of studies of psychological factors in Ménière's disease has focused on the role of stress as a possible cause of the illness or trigger of recurrent attacks. This line of inquiry includes investigations of personality traits and interactions between personality traits and stress in individuals with Ménière's disease. The first papers were single case studies or case series using psychoanalytic methods. Fowler and Zeckel[1] investigated a theory that symptoms such as vertigo were caused by psychological factors that slowed blood flow in the small vessels of end organs. To test this theory in Ménière's disease, they observed capillary flow in the conjunctiva using slit lamp magnification as a putative marker of blood flow in the labyrinth during active and quiescent phases of Ménière's disease in 23 patients. They theorized that their subjects' sexual inhibition or suppressed aggression manifested in episodes of interpersonal conflict and psychic agitation leading to sluggishness of circulation to the labyrinth, which they extrapolated from their measures of conjunctival capillaries. Their observations were not timed systematically with respect to subjects' external stressors or Ménière's symptoms and any link between conjunctival injection and labyrinthine blood flow would have been tenuous, at best. However, the concept that the central nervous system plays a role in the pathophysiologic mechanisms of Ménière's disease, via vascular, neural, or humoral influences, remains an area of active investigation to this day. Furthermore, the psychological profile of their 23 subjects revealed personality traits that were recognized again in subsequent studies, as noted below.

In cross-sectional surveys, 80% of Swedish[16] and Japanese[17] patients reported that external factors, such as stress at home or work, caused exacerbations of their Ménière's disease. However, prospective studies cast doubt on this widely held belief. Two studies followed patients with Ménière's disease over several months as they recorded symptoms and life events. Andersson, et al[2] had 20 subjects record symptoms of tinnitus, hearing loss, dizziness, Ménière's attacks, and stress on visual analog scales in daily diaries for an average of 194 days (range 45–351 days). A moving average time series analysis showed no consistent temporal pattern between perceived levels of stress and any of the core symptoms of Ménière's disease or Ménière's attacks for the study cohort as a whole. However, individual differences emerged. Seven (35%) subjects had positive correlations between self-reported stress levels and severity of at least two Ménière's symptoms. They reported increased stress on the day of increased symptoms, but not on the days before or after symptom exacerbations. Data from four (20%) subjects showed a relationship between stress and Ménière's attacks. Seven (35%) subjects had no correlation at all between stress and Ménière's symptoms or attacks. Time resolution in this study was one day, so it could not be determined within any given day if stress was a cause or consequence of Ménière's symptoms.

Soderman et al[3] followed 46 subjects with Ménière's disease for an average of 18 months. As soon as possible after the onset of an attack, subjects were asked to report mental, emotional, and physical stress from the previous 48 hours on a data collection form developed for the study. Mental stress was defined as "something that makes you mentally exhausted." Emotional stress was defined as a positive or negative events "that make you nervous, worried, or anxiety-ridden." Physical stress was defined as "something that demands your physical exertion to manage in time." After 22 days without an attack, subjects were asked to rate the previous 48 hours in an identical manner. The temporal resolution of this study was 1 hour, although it focused only on the time period before attacks. During the study period, 24 (52%) subjects had at least one attack, giving a total of 153 attacks and a larger number of comparison periods available for analysis. The authors reported that the relative risk of an attack within 3 hours of an emotional stress was 5.10 (95% CI = 2.37–10.98). The relative risk within 1 hour of a mental stress was 4.16 (95% CI = 1.46–11.83). Physical stress was not related to attacks. Salim et al[4] developed a new method to analyze these data and recalculated the relative risk of an attack within 140 minutes of an emotional stress as 3.33. These results would seem to support the theory that stress raises the risk of Ménière's attacks. However, a detailed examination of the results is much more informative than the risk ratios alone. Only 12 (8%) of 153 attacks from the entire cohort were preceded by emotional stress and those occurred in just 7 (29%) of the 24 subjects who had attacks, all of whom had at least 4 attacks during the study period. One subject had, by far, the largest number of attacks (29) and the largest number (4) preceded by emotional stress. No subject who experienced fewer than four attacks during the study period had an attack preceded by emotional stress. Mental stress was reported before just 5 (3%) attacks, all in different subjects. By comparison, Salim et al[4] used the same method to determine that the relative risk of an attack within 40 minutes of a sudden head movement was 77.4. Interestingly, at the time of study enrollment, 61% of subjects reported that stress triggered attacks. This rate of attribution was in line with the cross-sectional investigations of Hägnebo et al[16] and Takahashi et al,[17] but was not borne out by the prospective data.

The relative risk of emotional stress preceding a Ménière's attack is statistically significant, whether it is 5.10 as originally determined by Soderman et al[3] or 3.33 as recalculated by Salim et al.[4] Nevertheless, this risk must be put in proper perspective, both clinically and mechanistically. The absolute risk of emotional stress causing a Ménière's attack was low and that risk was confined to the fraction of patients with more frequent attacks.[3] Even in those individuals, emotional stress preceded a minority of attacks. The studies of Anderson et al,[2] Soderman et al,[3] and Salim et al[4] counter the commonly held belief that stress, in general, worsens the course of Ménière's disease. However, they do not exclude stress as a trigger of Ménière's symptoms for some patients at some times. The challenge is to identify the most vulnerable patients and most salient triggers.

The scientific impetus behind the studies of Ménière's disease and stress can be traced to the work of Holmes and Rahe[18] and others who developed what has been called the general stress model of illness. This model postulates that stress has an adverse effect on physical and emotional health by repeatedly activating the sympathetic nervous system and triggering the release of stress hormones in ways that are damaging to the organism. In recent years, the general stress model has been replaced by a concept of individual vulnerability and resiliency. According to this newer theory,[19] individuals have an inherent vulnerability to adverse life events that is genetically determined, but mitigated by protective factors, such as positive experiences and strong social support. Interactions between individual vulnerability and environment, both positive and negative, determine physical and mental health outcomes. This theory has spawned research on gene-environment interactions that may be much more informative about pathophysiologic mechanisms of illness and, eventually, may be used to individualize treatment selection. For example, a genetic polymorphism in the promoter region of the serotonin transporter gene (SLC6A4/5HTTLPR), which regulates the efficiency of serotonergic neurotransmission, has shown a modest,[20] but not universally detected,[21] association with major depression. The limited findings of these direct association studies stand in contrast to stronger results from gene-environment interaction studies involving the same gene. Cervilla et al[22] examined the interaction between 5HTTLPR genotype and exposure to adverse life events and found a strong genotype dependent, dose-response relationship between the number of traumatic events in subjects' lives and the likelihood of developing major depression. Subjects who possessed the previously identified vulnerable genotype ('s' allele) were susceptible to the onset of major depression after a single traumatic event, but those with more resilient genotypes were not likely to develop depression unless exposed to two or more serious events. The failure of published studies to show a global relationship between Ménière's disease and stress may be due to the fact that they were designed in accordance with the general stress model and, as such, did not consider variations in individual vulnerability. Future studies will have to account for individual vulnerability by measuring suspect genotypes or phenotypes in addition to objective measures of Ménière's disease state, not just self-reports of symptoms and stress levels. Adequately powered studies, constructed in this manner, should be able to shed more light on the long-standing question of a relationship between stress and the clinical course of Ménière's disease.

Published data are available to guide such investigations. Savastano and colleagues[23] observed a relationship between personality traits, perception of disease severity, and levels of anxiety and depression in a study of 50 Italian patients with Ménière's disease. Mean scores for neuroticism (ie, personality traits of pessimistic worry, internal tension, self-consciousness, and poor tolerance for stress) on the Eysenck Personality Inventory and psychological perception of disease on the Illness Behavior Questionnaire were higher than population norms for the study group as a whole. However, elevated scores were not normally distributed within the cohort. The largest subgroup of subjects had normal personality profiles, normal scores on the Illness Behavior Questionnaire, and normal ratings of anxiety and depression. A smaller subgroup had elevated scores on all measures. This group was somewhat older and had a longer duration of disease, but the authors concluded that personality traits, not physical factors of Ménière's disease, conferred individual vulnerability to the development of distressing illness beliefs, anxiety, and depression.

In two studies in Japan, Takahashi and colleagues[10,11] developed a questionnaire to measure Type A personality behaviors (eg, agitation, competitiveness, sense of time pressure, engrossment in work), social inhibition (self-consciousness, acquiescence to others), evasive behaviors (avoiding difficult tasks, blaming others), environmental stressors at home and work, somatic symptoms (vertigo, as well as nonspecific chest and abdominal complaints), and means of relaxation. They used this questionnaire to survey patients with Ménière's disease and two comparative populations. In their first study,[10] the authors compared 60 patients with Ménière's disease to 936 general medical outpatients. Patients with Ménière's disease had higher scores than the comparison group in all areas except use of relaxation. Among patients with Ménière's disease, the score for life stressors did not correlate with other scores, whereas it did in general medical outpatients. This could be due to the smaller size of the Ménière's group. However, the authors concluded that the results identified a link between agitated, driven, and socially inhibited personality traits, evasive behaviors, and somatic symptoms that is inherent in patients with Ménière's disease and not driven by external events. The second study[11] included 185 patients with Ménière's disease, 144 patients with low-frequency sensorineural hearing loss without vertigo, and 329 age- and sex-matched controls randomly selected from a pool of general medical outpatients. In addition to the questionnaire from the first study, the investigators tracked subjects' daily sleep, wake, and activity schedules. The three groups did not differ in daily schedules and there were no group differences among men or women regarding exposure to stressors, means of relaxation, or ratings of nonvertiginous physical symptoms. As in the first study, subjects with Ménière's disease, both men and women, had significantly higher scores for driven and inhibited personality traits than matched controls. The hearing loss group also differed from controls on these measures, but to not to the same extent as the Ménière's group. Taken together, these two studies found no differences between patients with Ménière's disease and comparison groups on exposure to external events, lifestyle or schedules, means of relaxation, or general psychosomatic symptoms. However, they found and confirmed higher levels of driven and inhibited personality traits in patients with Ménière's disease.

The results from Takahashi and colleagues[10,11] match the older studies of personality traits in patients with Ménière's disease that were mentioned above. Fowler and Zeckel[1] identified the traits of excessive tension, suppressed aggression, and competitive drive in their psychoanalytic study in the United States more than 50 years ago. Savastano et al[23] found increased neuroticism, which includes internal tension, suppressed hostility, and self-consciousness, in their Italian study. De Valck et al[12] had a somewhat different result. They investigated obsessiveness in patients with Ménière's disease by measuring conscientiousness using the NEO Five Factor Inventory in 108 Belgian patients with Ménière's disease or other vertiginous conditions (paroxysmal vertigo, vestibular neuronitis, acoustic neuroma). Conscientiousness embodies a sense of order, dutifulness, and striving for achievement, which are some of the traits identified in the previous studies. Conscientiousness scores were significantly higher than population norms in all patients with vertigo, but did not differ between those with Ménière's disease and other neurotologic illnesses. This suggests that the obsessive traits of dutifulness and engrossment in work may not be unique to patients with Ménière's' disease, but leaves open the possibility that other neurotic and introverted traits (eg, pessimistic worry, internal tension, suppressed aggression, and social inhibition) create a link between reactivity to stressful life events and Ménière's symptoms in some patients, possibly those who suffer frequent attacks or more persistent symptoms.

Psychiatric Disorders in Patients with Ménière's Disease

Anxiety and depression present another psychological challenge for patients with Ménière's disease and the clinicians who treat them. Kirby and Yardley[24] reviewed published research on psychological disturbances in patients with Ménière's disease. They identified 28 studies on this topic published between 1977 and 2004, only one of which was longitudinal in design. Fortunately, a few longitudinal studies on anxiety, depression, and quality of life in patients with Ménière's disease have been published since 2004, but most information about these topics is from cross-sectional studies of modest size. It is tempting to consider anxiety and depression to be "reasonable" responses to Ménière's disease, but this stance was rejected by Celestino et al.[25] Psychiatric illness is not a normal response to medical illness and many patients with Ménière's disease do not develop psychiatric comorbidity. However, recognition and treatment of psychiatric disorders, when they occur, are important steps to minimizing the total burden of illness borne by patients with Ménière's disease.

Early studies indicated that patients with Ménière's disease may be more likely to develop anxiety or depression than individuals with other neurotologic illnesses and that the prevalence of psychiatric morbidity may be related to the activity and severity of Ménière's symptoms. For example, Filipo et al[5] found that patients with Ménière's disease were more dysphoric than those with otosclerosis. They also found that patients with Ménière's disease who were treated surgically were more dysphoric, anxious, somatically preoccupied, and had higher levels of health anxiety than those who were treated medically. Presumably, patients who required surgical treatment had more severe illnesses than those who were treated medically. Coker et al[6] used two different self-reports and found that 32% to 39% of patients with inactive Ménière's disease and 70% to 80% of patients with active illness had clinically significant depressive symptoms. Soderman et al[7] identified more anxiety than depression in a cross-sectional study of 112 patients with Ménière's disease. Their subjects completed multiple self-reports to rate Ménière's symptoms, psychological status, and quality of life. Fifty-seven (51%) subjects had elevated scores on the anxiety subscale of the Hospital Anxiety and Depression Scale (HADS), whereas 17 (15%) had elevated scores on the depression subscale. In multiple regression analyses, the sense of coherence, which is a measure of the capacity to cope with stressful life circumstances, was the strongest predictor of emotional state as measured by the HADS. Celestino et al[25] found that the development of Ménière's disease worsened pre-existing anxiety disorders in some, but not all, patients. Other individuals developed new onset agoraphobia with or without panic after the onset of Ménière's symptoms. Kirby and Yardley[26] found that anxiety disorders were most common in patients who feared the uncertainty of future Ménière's attacks.

The most recent studies of psychiatric morbidity in Ménière's disease have employed psychiatric diagnostic examinations of patients and control populations. Eckhardt-Henn et al[8] investigated the prevalence of psychiatric comorbidity in patients with several neurotologic illnesses. The rates of active psychiatric illnesses, mostly anxiety and depressive disorders, were substantially higher in patients with Ménière's disease (57%) and vestibular migraine (65%) than in patients with vestibular neuronitis (22%), benign paroxysmal positional vertigo (15%), or control subjects (20%). The odds ratios for anxiety disorders in patients with Ménière's disease (38.7) and vestibular migraine (26.6) were strikingly high. This study was methodologically sound with detailed neurotologic and psychiatric examinations of all subjects, but the total study population was small ($N = 68$), including only seven patients with Ménière's disease. There were no correlations between neurotologic and psychometric variables leading the authors to conclude that the link between anxiety, depression, and neurotologic illness, particularly in patients with Ménière's disease and vestibular migraine, reflected the existence of premorbid personality characteristics.[27] In a year-long follow-up study,[9] the investigators found that the strongest predictor of patients developing a psychiatric disorder after the onset of a neurotologic illness, including Ménière's disease, was a history of psychiatric illness predating the onset of vertigo.

A few studies have attempted to link biological markers of stress and depression to Ménière's disease.[28–29] The circadian rhythms of hormones such as cortisol and melatonin are altered in a portion of patients with major depression. Aoki et al[28] found that the circadian secretion of melatonin was phase advanced and blunted in patients with Ménière's disease relative to controls. Patients with Ménière's disease also had higher depression and stress scores than controls, but there were no correlations between melatonin secretion, depression, and exposure to stressful life events. In another study, Aoki et al[29] identified elevations of vasopressin (a stress hormone) in patients with Ménière's disease during acute attacks of vertigo. As was the case with alterations in melatonin, however, this finding was not related to levels of depression or stress. Abnormalities of cortisol secretion have been linked to hippocampal atrophy in patients with posttraumatic stress disorder. Van Cruijsen et al[30] searched for a similar effect in Ménière's disease, but found no differences in hippocampal volume between 10 patients with Ménière's disease and 10 controls with similar rating of daily stress and salivary cortisol levels. In all three studies the total number of subjects was small (eg, 19 in the melatonin study), so the negative results may reflect underpowered investigations and Type II errors.

In summary, the prevalence of anxiety and depressive disorders is increased in patients with Ménière's disease relative to control subjects. Psychiatric illness is not simply a reaction to Ménière's disease, because neurotologic parameters do not correlate with the prevalence or severity of anxiety or depression. Rather, a portion of patients with Ménière's disease appears to be vulnerable to developing psychiatric morbidity. Pre-existing psychiatric illness is a risk factor, although not all patients with psychiatric histories experience a worsening of their mental health and some patients develop de novo psychiatric disorders after the onset of Ménière's symptoms.

Quality of Life in Patients with Ménière's Disease

Yardley et al[31] surveyed members of a Ménière's self-help group by mail. Not surprisingly, poorer quality of life was related to more severe vertigo, hearing loss, tinnitus, and pressure in the ear. Nonotologic factors associated with poorer quality of life included younger age, female sex, living alone, lower occupational status, and belief that the otologist was not helpful. In a separate study, Holgers and Finizia[32] also found that tinnitus severity had a significant negative effect on health related quality of life, but 40% of the variance in perceived tinnitus severity was related to emotional factors. Soderman et al[33] found a positive relationship between sense of coherence (ie, capacity to cope with stressful life circumstances) and better quality of life in patients with Ménière's disease. Thus, quality of life for patients with Ménière's disease is affected by positive and negative physical and psychological variables. This suggests that quality of life may be enhanced by a comprehensive treatment plan that optimizes control of physical symptoms, addresses psychiatric illness, and enhances innate coping skills. This assumption has not been subjected to systematic inquiry.

Positive Psychological Responses to Ménière's Disease

The psychosocial effects of Ménière's disease are not entirely negative. Individuals with other chronic or life threatening conditions (eg, HIV/AIDS, malignancies) have reported a number of positive developments, such as better organized priorities in life, improved relationships with family members and friends, and greater empathy for others who are sick. Stephens et al[34] investigated the possibility that individuals with Ménière's disease might have similar, positive experiences. They surveyed 272 members of the Finnish Ménière Federation by mail, receiving 181 responses. Included in the questionnaire were validated measures of

Ménière's symptoms, activity restrictions, sense of coherence, and quality of life, plus two open-ended questions about positive experiences that followed an introductory paragraph explaining that some individuals describe positive aspects of being ill. Seventy-five percent of respondents listed at least one positive experience. Responses to the two questions were analyzed with qualitative methods. Six themes emerged: personal development (ie, broadened perspective on life), leisure, lifestyle, and general health (positive comments from some subjects on ability to keep working and from others on enjoying leisure activities after cutting back on work), understanding of illness (eg, symptoms not always present and not lethal), disease-specific comments (eg, individual management strategies), interpersonal relationships (closer connections to family members and friends), and camaraderie of the Ménière Federation. Respondents with higher quality of life scores were more likely to make positive comments. Symptom severity ratings were not associated with likelihood of a positive response. These themes were echoed in a study of 301 members of the Ménière's Society UK who reported positive change in the domains of appreciation of life, relating to others, personal strength, new possibilities, and spiritual change on the Posttraumatic Growth Inventory.[35] During 10 months of involvement in the self-help group, social comparisons with others in the group affected change. Individuals who made positive social comparisons adjusted better to their illness, whereas those who made negative social comparisons had poorer adjustments.[36]

Treatment of Psychiatric Morbidity in Patients with Ménière's Disease

There have been no systematic studies of psychopharmacologic or psychotherapeutic treatments specifically for patients with Ménière's disease. Three open label clinical trials of selective serotonin reuptake inhibitor (SSRI) antidepressants for patients with chronic dizziness included subjects with Ménière's disease,[13–15] although the entry criteria for each of these studies was chronic dizziness, not episodic vertigo. Patients with Ménière's disease appeared to tolerate SSRI antidepressants as well as other patients despite the fact that all drugs in this class list dizziness as a potential adverse effect. Clinical experience suggests that these medications are effective for treating coexisting anxiety and depressive disorders in patients with Ménière's disease and do not interfere with medical therapies for Ménière's disease, itself, or with vestibular rehabilitation.

Yardley and Kirby[37] tested the efficacy of a community educational intervention in 360 patients with Ménière's disease. They mailed educational booklets to two groups of 120 patients. A third group of 120 patients served as a control. The booklet mailed to the first group instructed recipients in home-based vestibular rehabilitation techniques. The booklet mailed to the second group contained information on applied relaxation techniques, cognitive reframing of negative beliefs about the disease, and tips on lifestyle modification strategies, all designed to reduce anxiety. After 3 months, the vestibular rehabilitation group reported reduced physical symptoms, lower anxiety, less disability, and fewer negative beliefs about dizziness. The applied relaxation group reported less disability. The control group did not improve. After 6 months, nearly 40% of recipients in both intervention groups reported overall improvement in morbidity compared to only 15% of the control group, including significantly greater ability to understand and cope with symptoms. Adherence rates to self-treatment suggestions were low, but positively correlated to the outcomes of this simple and inexpensive intervention.

Effects of Psychological Factors on Medical and Surgical Treatments for Ménière's Disease

A few studies indicate that psychological factors may affect outcomes of medical or surgical treatments for Ménière's disease. Willatt and Yung[38] reported that patients who experienced persistent unsteadiness after labyrinthectomy were more likely to be anxious and/or depressed, have an external health locus of control (ie, a belief that factors beyond their control determined their health), work in sedentary jobs, and have extraverted personalities. The reason for a negative outcome in extraverted patients is not clear, as most research has linked Ménière's disease to introverted personality traits.

Two groups of investigators examined the influence of pretreatment functioning on post-treatment outcomes using the 1995 American Academy of Otolaryngology-Head and Neck Surgery Functional Level Scale (FLS) for Ménière's disease. Tyagi et al[39] investigated changes in functional outcomes after endolymphatic sac decompression surgery in 39 patients who completed retrospective questionnaires at a mean of 29 months after surgery. They reported excellent outcomes in their cohort as a whole, with 82% of subjects achieving class A vertigo control. However, preoperative FLS scores affected outcome. All patients with preoperative scores of 4 or higher benefited from surgery, but none of those with preoperative scores of 3 or lower were helped by sac decompression. A floor effect may have limited the authors' ability to show benefits for subjects with lower preoperative scores, but the risk benefit ratio of surgical intervention appeared to favor those who were more functionally impaired before operation.

Boleas-Agguirre et al[40] performed a more detailed assessment of functional and psychological outcomes in 103 patients who were followed prospectively after treatment with transtympanic gentamicin. They, too, achieved excellent results with 81% of patients free of vertigo spells at a mean of 5.3 years after treatment. At study endpoint, none of the subjects reported vertigo attacks during the previous 6 months. Their findings regarding the effect of pretreatment FLS scores on post-treatment outcomes were more nuanced than the smaller, retrospective study of Tyagi et al.[39] Boleas-Agguirre et al[40] found that subjects with pretreatment FLS scores of 6 had poor outcomes. Examination of their data showed that high anxiety distinguished these subjects from those with lower scores. Patients with pretreatment FLS scores of 3, 4, or 5 had mean somatic anxiety scores ranging from 15 to 20 on the Vertigo Symptom Scale (VSS), whereas patients with pretreatment scores of 6 had a mean somatic anxiety score of 35. Moreover, 16 (15.5%) subjects reported chronic unsteadiness after treatment. This group of patients had no pre- to post-treatment reductions in scores on the UCLA-Dizziness Questionnaire or Dizziness Handicap Inventory physical or functional subscales. Their VSS somatic anxiety scores did not improve either. The authors concluded that patients with FLS scores of 6 require unspecified "special care." What their data show is that these patients require proper attention to their anxiety.

Summary

Published research on the psychological attributes of Ménière's disease includes too few longitudinal studies of adequate size. Treatment research is quite sparse. Despite these limitations, there are important consistencies across studies from different eras and different theoretical frameworks. External stress is believed by most patients to trigger symptoms of Ménière's disease, but prospective studies have not upheld this conviction. Only the minority of patients with frequent spells seems to be vulnerable to emotional stress as a trigger of attacks. Studies spanning 50 years and three continents suggest that tense, driven, and self-inhibited personality traits are more common in patients with Ménière's disease than general medical outpatients. These traits may link stress vulnerability to greater physical morbidity in some individuals with Ménière's disease, but this hypothesis is yet to be tested. Anxiety and depression are common in patients with Ménière's disease. Individuals may be predisposed to behavioral comorbidity by psychiatric illness that predates Ménière's symptoms, but anxiety and depression also develop de novo after onset of the disease. Anxiety has a negative effect on functional levels in patients with Ménière's disease and may exert an adverse effect on outcomes of common medical and surgical treatments. There are no controlled studies of interventions for psychological morbidity in Ménière's disease. A few open trials of anxiolytic antidepressants (SSRIs) for chronic dizziness have included patients with Ménière's disease. These extremely limited data, plus clinical experience, suggest that anxiety and depression can be adequately treated in patients with Ménière's disease, resulting in improved physical and mental outcomes. Finally, Ménière's disease, like other serious illnesses, may be an impetus for psychological growth, prompting individuals to reorganize their priorities in life, develop better relationships with family members and friends, and have greater empathy for the suffering of others.

References

1. Fowler EP, Zeckel A. Psychophysiological factors in Ménière's disease. *Psychosom Med.* 1953;15:127–139.
2. Andersson G, Hägnebo C, Yardley L. Stress and symptoms of Ménière's disease: a time-series analysis. *J Psychosom Res.* 1997;43:595–603.
3. Söderman AC, Möller J, Bagger-Sjöbäck D, Bergenius J, Hallqvist J. Stress as a trigger of attacks in Ménière's disease.

A case-crossover study. *Laryngoscope.* 2004;114:1843–1848.
4. Salim A, Becker NG, Möller J, Hessén-Söderman AC. An analysis for a cross-over cohort study with an application to the study of triggers of Menière's disease. *Stat Med.* 2007;26:1136–1149.
5. Filipo R, Lazzari R, Barbara M, Franzese A, Petruzzellis MC. Psychologic evolution of patients with Ménière's disease in relation to therapy. *Am J Otol.* 1988; 9:306–309.
6. Coker NJ, Coker RR, Jenkins HA, Vincent KR. Psychological profile of patients with Ménière's disease. *Arch Otolaryngol Head Neck Surg.* 1989;115:1355–1357.
7. Soderman AC, Bagger-Sjoback D, Bergenius J, Langius A. Factors influencing quality of life in patients with Ménière's disease, identified by a multidimensional approach. *Otol Neurotol.* 2002;23: 941–948.
8. Eckhardt-Henn A, Best C, Bense S, et al. Psychiatric comorbidity in different organic vertigo syndromes. *J Neurol.* 2008;255:420–428.
9. Best C, Eckhardt-Henn A, Tschan R, Dieterich M. Psychiatric morbidity and comorbidity in different vestibular vertigo syndromes: results of a prospective longitudinal study over one year. *J Neurol.* 2009;256:58–65.
10. Takahashi M, Ishida K, Iida M, Yamashita H, Sugawara K. Analysis of lifestyle and behavioral characteristics in Ménière's disease patients and a large control population. *Acta Otolaryngol.* 2001;201:254–256.
11. Onuki J, Takahashi M, Odagiri K, Wada R, Sato R. Comparative study of the daily lifestyle of patients with Ménière's disease and controls. *Ann Otol Rhinol Laryngol.* 2005;114:927–933.
12. De Valck CF, Wuyts FL, Vanspauwen R, Walravens S, Van de Heyning PH. Conscientiousness in patients with Ménière's disease. *Otol Neurotol.* 2007;28:365–368.
13. Horii A, Mitani K, Kitahara T, Uno A, Takeda N, Kubo T. Paroxetine, a selective serotonin reuptake inhibitor, reduces depressive symptoms and subjective handicaps in patients with dizziness. *Otol Neurotol.* 2004;25:536–543.
14. Horii A, Uno A, Kitahara T, et al. Effects of fluvoxamine on anxiety, depression, and subjective handicaps of chronic dizziness patients with or without neuro-otologic diseases. *J Vestib Res.* 2007;17:1–8.
15. Staab JP, Ruckenstein MJ, Solomon D, Shepard NT. Serotonin reuptake inhibitors for dizziness with psychiatric symptoms. *Arch Otolaryngol Head Neck Surg.* 2002;128:554–560.
16. Hägnebo C, Melin L, Larsen HC, Lindberg P, Lyttkens L, Scott B. The influence of vertigo, hearing impairment and tinnitus on the daily life of Ménière patients. *Scand Audiol.* 1997;26:69–76.
17. Takahashi M, Odagiri K, Sato R, Wada R, Onuki J. Personal factors involved in onset or progression of Ménière's disease and low-tone sensorineural hearing loss. *ORL J Otorhinolaryngol Relat Spec.* 2005;67:300–304.
18. Rahe RH, Meyer M, Smith M, Kjaer G, Holmes T. Social stress and illness onset. *J Psychosom Res.* 1964;54:35–44.
19. Gonda X, Fountoulakis KN, Juhasz G, et al. Association of the s allele of the 5-HTTLPR with neuroticism-related traits and temperaments in a psychiatrically healthy population. *Eur Arch Psychiatry Clin Neurosci.* 2009;259:106–113.
20. Eley TC, Sugden K, Corsico A, et al. Gene-environment interaction analysis of serotonin system markers with adolescent depression. *Mol Psychiatry.* 2004; 9:908–915.
21. Mendlewicz J, Massat I, Souery D, et al. Serotonin transporter 5HTTLPR polymorphism and affective disorders: no evidence of association in a large European multicenter study. *Eur J Hum Genet.* 2004;12:377–382.
22. Cervilla JA, Molina E, Rivera M, et al. The risk for depression conferred by stressful life events is modified by variation at the serotonin transporter 5HTTLPR

genotype: evidence from the Spanish PREDICT-Gene cohort. *Mol Psychiatry.* 2007;12:748–755.
23. Savastano M, Maron MB, Mangialaio M, Longhi P, Rizzardo R. Illness behaviour, personality traits, anxiety, and depression in patients with Ménière's disease. *J Otolaryngol.* 1996;25:329–333.
24. Kirby SE, Yardley L. Understanding psychological distress in Ménière's disease: a systematic review. *Psychol Health Med.* 2008;13:257–273.
25. Celestino D, Rosini E, Carucci ML, Marconi PL, Vercillo E. Ménière's disease and anxiety disorders. *Acta Otorhinolaryngol Ital.* 2003;23:421–427.
26. Kirby SE, Yardley L. Cognitions associated with anxiety in Ménière's disease. *J Psychosom Res.* 2009;66:111–118.
27. Best C, Eckhardt-Henn A, Diener G, Bense S, Breuer P, Dieterich M. Interaction of somatoform and vestibular disorders. *J Neurol Neurosurg Psychiatry.* 2006;77:658–664.
28. Aoki M, Asai M, Nishihori T, Mizuta K, Ito Y, Ando K. The relevance of an elevation in the plasma vasopressin levels to the pathogenesis of Ménière's attack. *J Neuroendocrinol.* 2007;19:901–906.
29. Aoki M, Yokota Y, Hayashi T, et al. Disorder of the saliva melatonin circadian rhythm in patients with Ménière's disease. *Acta Neurol Scand.* 2006;113: 256–261.
30. Van Cruijsen N, Hiemstra WM, Meiners LC, Wit HP, Albers FW. Hippocampal volume measurement in patients with Ménière's disease: a pilot study. *Acta Otolaryngol.* 2007;127:1018–1023.
31. Yardley L, Dibb B, Osborne G. Factors associated with quality of life in Ménière's disease. *Clin Otolaryngol Allied Sci.* 2003;28:436–441.
32. Holgers KM, Finizia C. Health profiles for patients with Ménière's disease. *Noise Health.* 2001;4:71–80.
33. Soderman AC, Bergenius J, Bagger-Sjoback D, Tjell C, Langius A. Patients' subjective evaluations of quality of life related to disease-specific symptoms, sense of coherence, and treatment in Ménière's disease. *Otol Neurotol.* 2001; 22:526–533.
34. Stephens D, Kentala E, Varpa K, Pyykkö. Positive experiences associated with Ménière's disorder. *Otol Neurotol.* 2007; 28:982–987.
35. Dibb B. Positive change with Ménière's disease. *Br J Health Psychol.* 2009;14(pt 4): 613–624.
36. Dibb B, Yardley L. How does social comparison within a self-help group influence adjustment to chronic illness? A longitudinal study. *Soc Sci Med.* 2006; 63:1602–1613.
37. Yardley L, Kirby S. Evaluation of booklet-based self-management of symptoms in Ménière's disease: a randomized controlled trial. *Psychosom Med.* 2006;68: 762–769.
38. Willatt DJ, Yung MW. Prognostic factors in labyrinthectomy. *J Laryngol Otol.* 1988;102:785–787.
39. Tyagi I, Goyal A, Syal R. Sac surgery results as a function of preoperative distress level. *Otol Neurotol.* 2006;27:951–955.
40. Boleas-Aguirre MS, Sánchez-Ferrandiz N, Guillén-Grima F, Perez N. Long-term disability of class A patients with Ménière's disease after treatment with intratympanic gentamicin. *Laryngoscope.* 2007;117:1474–1481.

14

Challenging Cases

Michael J. Ruckenstein

This book has sought to emphasize an evidence-based approach to treatment of patients with Ménière's disease. That said, as described in Chapter 10 on medical treatment, we do not have a medication that specifically addresses the underlying disease state. All medications used to date seem to evoke a nonspecific or placebo type response in patients. Vestibular suppressants can suppress the underlying vertigo; however, they cannot prevent attacks and, therefore, will only mitigate symptoms of vertigo when they occur. Chronic use of vestibular suppressants should, except in specific cases, be discouraged as they prevent vestibular compensation.

Surgical interventions that do provide excellent vertigo control have evolved. However, all surgeries that offer treatment results that exceed what can be expected from a placebo intervention involve ablating the vestibular system in the affected ear. Thus, their utilization has to be approached with caution particularly in certain patients, such as those with bilateral disease. The result is that the treatment of Ménière's disease is currently both an art and a science. Physicians have to make judicious use of the treatments that are nonspecific in their treatment effects. In addition, careful consideration must be given to the differential diagnosis to ensure that the patient is indeed suffering from vertigo secondary to Ménière's disease.

The following cases emphasize diagnostic and therapeutic challenges to the treating physician. There probably is no absolutely correct way to manage these cases. I offer a treatment algorithm that I have found useful in my practice. Due to the small numbers of these patients, it is difficult to arrive on an evidence-based solution for these problems.

Case 1. Migrainous Vertigo Versus Ménière's Disease

A 42-year-old female presents with a recurrent history of vertigo that began during her teenage years. The vertigo typically lasts for minutes to hours and is associated with nausea and vomiting. At its onset, the vertigo occurred very infrequently. She only had two or three episodes vertigo throughout her teenage years and early 20s. At age 25, she experienced a significant loss of hearing in her right ear. The hearing loss did not fluctuate and has remained stable since its onset. Recently, she has had an exacerbation in her episodes of vertigo. They are now occurring either weekly or biweekly. They last for hours and are quite disabling. There is no fluctuation in hearing. She was diagnosed with migraine headaches while in university in her 20s. She uses abortive therapy for the migraine headaches. The migraine headaches do not occur with the vertigo. She has approximately three or four severe migraines a year that do respond to the abortive treatments. There is a strong family history of migraines on her maternal side. Other than that, she carries no risk factors in her personal or family history for inner ear or vestibular disease.

Her physical examination was within normal limits. The only abnormality noted was a Weber test that lateralized to the left ear. Audiometric assessment revealed a flat sensorineural hearing loss affecting the right ear with thresholds of between 50 and 60 decibels. Balance function tests show evidence of a right peripheral loss on calorics. There is residual vestibular function in both ears. MRI scan showed no lesions of the VIIIth nerve or temporal bone and was read as normal.

The dilemma that this patient poses is whether her vertigo results from Ménière's disease or from migraines. The episodes of vertigo are consistent with both diagnoses. She does have hearing loss but the hearing in the right ear does not fluctuate. Thus, there is no evidence on history, examination, or testing of active disease affecting her right ear. The headaches are not coincident with the vertigo; however, this is commonly the case in patients with migrainous vertigo. Thus, the history, examination, and testing do not provide us with any strong evidence that would allow us to favor one diagnosis over the other.

The general treatment strategy I employ in these patients is to attempt to rule out migrainous vertigo as an etiology. It is important **not** to proceed with vestibuloablative treatment immediately in these patients. This could cause an unfortunate vestibular loss and a poor therapeutic outcome if the patient is truly suffering from migrainous vertigo. Thus, initially, I would recommend that the patient address migraine prophylaxis. This would include avoidance of migraine triggers. A migraine prophylaxin should be administered as a therapeutic trial. Drugs to be considered for this include acetazolamide either 250 mg BID to TID or the extended release form (Diamox–CR®) at a dose of 500 mg, one pill, once to twice a day. Acetazolamide has been shown to benefit some patients with migrainous vertigo as noted in Chapter 10. Other options would include nortriptyline given at a dose initiating at 10 mg QHS and increasing on a weekly basis by 10 mg up to 50 mg QHS. Topramate currently is a popular migraine prophylaxin. This is given at a dose of 25 mg at night for one week then increasing by 25 mg a day every week to a maximum of 200 mg per day. The therapeutic range is fairly wide in this drug. Patients often complain of side effects including cognitive dysfunction.

I would usually recommend a 1- to 2-month trial of a migraine prophylaxin and see how the patient's vertigo responds. If the patient responds with good vertigo control, then it is reasonable to conclude that he or she is suffering from migrainous vertigo and I would recommend continuing this medication regimen. If, however, the vertigo persisted despite an adequate therapeutic trial, then I would consider it must more likely that the patient is suffering from Ménière's disease. Treatment options at that point include administration of a diuretic such as Dyazide or proceeding to a vestibular ablative procedure such as intratympanic gentamicin treatment.

Case 2. Bilateral Ménière's Disease

A 67-year-old male presents with a long history of Ménière's disease. He first experienced right-sided hearing loss in his 20s. This hearing loss was associated with episodes of true rotatory vertigo lasting for hours. He was managed conservatively with diuretics, vasodilators, and a low-salt diet. He underwent a right endolymphatic shunt procedure in his 40s. He continued on the medical regimen and was doing reasonably well until he hit his 50s when he began developing increased hearing loss in his left ear. This, too, was associated with vertigo. The vertigo was controlled with vestibular suppressants, low-salt diet, and diuretic therapy. He ultimately underwent an endolymphatic shunt surgery on the left ear when he was 55 years old. He did well for several years but the vertigo resumed, occurring once every 2 to 3 months. At that point he was not experiencing fluctuation in hearing in either ear. Recently, the vertigo increased in frequency, occurring every 2 weeks. He wears bilateral hearing aids and is on a low-salt diet and a potassium-sparing diuretic. He uses a combination of meclizine and diazepam for vertigo control of acute episodes of vertigo.

His examination was significant for his being unable to perform tandem gate testing with eyes closed. He turned to the right on the Fukuda stepping test. The remainder of the exam was normal.

Audiometric assessment shows a flat sensorineural hearing loss in the right ear with thresholds of between 60 and 70 dB. Pure-tone audiometric assessment in the left ear shows thresholds of between 60 dB in the lower frequencies to 40 dB in the higher frequencies. Balance function tests show evidence of bilateral vestibular loss on caloric testing and rotatory chair testing. There is evidence of residual vestibular function in both ears. MRI scan showed no lesions of the VIIIth nerve or temporal bone. Serologic and immunologic testing were normal.

Treatment of patients with a bilateral Ménière's disease associated with a bilateral vestibular loss is a true challenge for several reasons. It often is difficult to ascertain which of the two affected ears is causing the acute symptoms of vertigo. Fluctuations in hearing in one ear coincident with the vertigo can identify the active ear. However, patients often cannot point to an active ear.

Therapeutic options for these patients are quite limited. In general, vestibular ablative therapy should be avoided so as to prevent exacerbating a bilateral vestibular loss and creating a disabling Dandy's syndrome with oscillopsia. This is extraordinarily debilitating to a patient and should be avoided at all costs. Nonspecific treatments, such as the Menniet device can be tried; however, my experience is that these more aggressive cases of Ménière's disease respond poorly to a nonspecific therapy. Intramuscular streptomycin treatment largely has been abandoned due to the difficulties in obtaining streptomycin and in titering the dose. On the rare occasion when it is absolutely clear which ear is causing the active disease, a low dose of intratympanic gentamicin can be given to try to stabilize that ear. In these situations, I would give one single dose of intratympanic gentamicin and test the patient's vestibular function 2 weeks subsequent to the treatment. If there has been a decline in vestibular function, I would stop treatment at that point in hopes that this would be sufficient ablation to control the vertigo. That said, I only have used this treatment option rarely in very specific and selective patients. More commonly, this is the one situation in which I will use chronic vestibular suppression to try to control the vertigo. I have had the most success in using the benzodiazepine clonazepam at doses of between 0.5 mg to 1 mg twice or three times a day. The patient generally slowly increases the dose from 0.5 mg to 1 mg and from twice to three times a day until the vertigo symptoms are controlled. This drug can be used for long periods of time and does not seem to lose efficacy. It certainly is not an ideal treatment but it is proven to be effective and fairly benign in this difficult-to-treat patient population.

Case 3. Ménière's Disease Versus Autoimmune Inner Ear Disease

A 29-year-old male presents with sudden right-sided unilateral sensorineural hearing loss.. The hearing loss is primarily in the low frequencies. He is placed on a 1-week course of prednisone and on the third day the hearing returns to normal levels. He completes the 1-week course of prednisone and does well for 2 weeks at which time the hearing loss recurs. At this point it, is associated with one episode of vertigo lasting for one hour. Prednisone is again prescribed but this time at higher doses for a total of 2 weeks. Seven days post-onset of the symptoms, the hearing loss again resolves. He does well for 2 months and again presents with low-frequency right–sided sensorineural hearing loss. His examination is significant only for tuning fork that lateralizes to the left ear. Audiometric assessment confirms low-frequency right–sided sensorineural loss with thresholds of approximately 50 to 60 dB in the affected frequencies. Balance function tests are within normal limits as is the MRI scan. Serologic and immunologic testing including a broad panel of tests for autoimmune disease all of which are negative.

This patient presents a dilemma as to whether he is suffering from Ménière's disease or autoimmune inner ear disease. Superficially, he appears to be responding to steroid treatment; however, these responses may be independent of the administered steroid and simply reflect the spontaneous fluctuations associated with Ménière's disease. Clearly, before committing a patient to long-term immunosuppression, it is prudent to try to confirm a diagnosis of autoimmune inner ear disease. Unfortunately, the only way to confirm the diagnosis is to demonstrate a positive response to steroids. Patients with completely normal immunologic testing can manifest steroid-responsive hearing loss, particularly if the testing has been performed subsequent to the administration of prednisone or similar immunosuppressants.

My general approach to these patients is to withhold prednisone therapy for a week or two after the onset of the hearing loss. There is generally a window of 14 days during which time the ear remains responsive to immunosuppression in cases of autoimmune disease. If the patient develops a spontaneous recovery of his hearing during this interval, then it is most likely that he is suffering from Ménière's disease and would not benefit from prolonged immunosuppression. If the hearing remains down after the 2 weeks, then I would readminister the prednisone at a dose of 60 mg a day for 2 weeks. If there is a positive therapeutic response, I would proceed with a very slow taper of prednisone over the course of a month and involve a rheumatologist in his care for management of immunosuppressant agents. If there is no response to the 60 mg of prednisone over a 2-week interval, I would taper the medication over the course of 10 days and consider him not responsive to immunosuppression. I would then continue to treat him as a patient with Ménière's disease. Particularly because the disease is at this point unilateral, I feel this is the most prudent course to prevent the patient being placed on long-term medication that carries significant side effects. The management algorithm would not change even if the patient did have some abnormalities on immunologic testing, given that these tests lack both sensitivity and specificity and, therefore, do not, in and of themselves, confirm a diagnosis of autoimmune inner ear disease. If, however, there are significant abnormalities on autoimmune testing, such as very high ANA titer, then I would work with a rheumatologist for evaluation of possible systemic autoimmune disease. I would institute immunosuppressive therapy if the patient manifested progressive hearing loss and if he or she demonstrated a clinical response.

15

Future Directions

Michael J. Ruckenstein, MD

Introduction

This book has explored an evidence-based approach to the analysis of Ménière's disease. As such, data pertaining to the pathophysiology and treatment of the disorder have been subjected to a rigid and critical analysis. The outcome of this analysis highlights the fact that many questions still exist regarding the entity we refer to as Ménière's disease.

Pathophysiology

The core of this book is Chapter 3 on pathophysiology. As described in Chapter 3, we really do not have an understanding as to the underlying pathophysiologic mechanisms responsible for Ménière's disease. The evidence points to the fact that endolymphatic hydrops, long associated with the disorder, is most likely an epiphenomenon and not the direct pathophysiologic mechanism responsible for the symptoms associated with Ménière's disease. As such, a complete re-examination of the pathophysiologic mechanisms responsible for Ménière's disease is required. Certainly, such mechanisms must include the generation of endolymphatic hydrops, as this finding is present in all temporal bones derived from patients with Ménière's disease. However, a paradigm shift is required in our approach to studying Ménière's disease if any progress is to be made regarding the understanding of the disorder.

Based on the current level of scientific research, it is my opinion that major advances in understanding of the pathophysiology of Ménière's disease will result from molecular biology experiments performed on patients with Ménière's disease. Unless we have some clue as to what the underlying process governing Ménière's disease is, an animal model that realistically mimics Ménière's disease is unlikely to be generated. However, if molecular biologic experiments can point to defects in patients with Ménière's disease, for example, abnormalities in channels, regulatory proteins, neurotransmission, then an animal model could be generated to better study the disorder. The rapid expansion of genetic and other molecular biologic techniques offers hope that the pathophysiology of the disorder will be elucidated one day in the near future.

Treatment

Unless the pathophysiology is better elucidated, it is highly unlikely we will develop any specific treatments for the disorder. At present, our treatments recruit either nonspecific or placebo type mechanisms or seek to eliminate symptoms by ablating vestibular function. I suspect that one day, we will look back at these treatments as being quite primitive. That day will come when the pathophysiology is better understood. Only at that time can treatments designed to address the underlying pathology be developed.

We hope that this text will provide a framework and food for thought when researching in the area of Ménière's disease. If that is its only success, then it will have been a very productive effort indeed!

Index

D

E

N

O

P

R

S